RADIATION SAFETY AND POSITIONING ANIMALS WITH ROPE AND TAPE IN VETERINARY RADIOGRAPHY

Matt Wright, DVM MS DACVR
Deon Spencer, RVT
Candi Stafford, RVT
Elizabeth Filed, ARRT

Copyright © 2013
Breedfreak, Inc.

All rights reserved. This book is protected by copyright. No part of this book may be reproduced in any form or by any means, including photocopying, or utilized by any information storage and retrieval system without written permission from the copyright owner.

Accurate indications, adverse reactions, and dosage schedules for drugs are provided in this book, but it is possible that they may change. The reader is urged to review the package information data of the manufacturers of the medications mentioned.

ISBN: 978-1-494-23935-0

CONTENTS

Introduction 5

CHAPTER 1
A (very) Short Guide to Radiation Safety for the Veterinary Technician 7

PART 1: Basic Radiation Safety 8
    Units, units, units 9
    Ionization; the good, the bad, the ugly 10
    Time, Distance, Shielding 13
    How much is too much? 15
    Putting things in Perspective – What do these doses mean to me? (*This is important – don't skim this part*) 16
    Personnel Monitoring Devices (a.k.a Film Badges) 18

PART 2: Radiation Safety for the Pregnant Worker 20
    Radiation Safety is Just Different for the Pregnant Employee 20
    Do this if you are pregnant or think you are pregnant 22

PART 3: Creating a Veterinary Radiographic Technique Chart 23
    An Example Technique Chart 27

PART 4: Special Considerations for Digital Radiography 30
    Ways to decrease noise and prevent dose creep: 33

PART 5: Common Sedation Protocols for Veterinary Radiography 35

PART 6: Two Charts to Print out and Post on the Wall 37

PART 7: Equipment you will need to non-manually restrain your patients 42

PART 8: Technical Basics of Positioning Patients for Radiography 45

Abdominal Radiographs 46
Thoracic Radiographs 47
Extremity Radiographs 49
Spinal Radiographs 50
Skull Radiographs 53

CHAPTER 2
Positioning with Sandbags, Rope, and Tape 61
    Lateral Thorax or Lateral Abdomen of the Dog 63
    Lateral Thorax or Lateral Abdomen Cat 64
    Ventral Dorsal Radiographs of the Thorax or Abdomen
    of the Cat 65
    Neck Radiography 67
    Pelvic Radiography of the Dog 69
    Ventral Dorsal Body and Pelvic Radiography of the Cat 73
    Lateral Radiographs of the Dog Stifle or Tarsal Joint 74
    Radiographs of the Cat Elbow Joint 76
    Lateral Radiographs of the Dog Elbow Joint 78
    Lateral Radiographs of the Dog Carpal Joint 80
    Lateral Radiographs of the Dog Shoulder Joint 82
    Radiographs of the Cat Paw 84

Appendix 1 85
Appendix 2 99

Introduction

Welcome to the Wonderful World of Safety, Sandbags, Rope, and Tape

A technician (who likes to rhyme) once said sandbags and tape keep you safe. She was convinced that hand holding patients for radiography was not appropriate and patients could be effectively restrained with sandbags, rope, tape, and sedation when necessary. She was right. Animals can be effectively restrained without unnecessarily exposing technical staff to ionizing radiation during radiography.

Restraining pets for radiography without holding them will prevent support staff from being bit, scratched, and maimed. It will also reduce their exposure to ionizing radiation.

All veterinary support staff should understand the basics of radiation safety. The goal of this book is to give veterinary support staff the knowledge necessary to understand why ionizing radiation can be harmful and what they can do to be safe while working with ionizing radiation.

The topics included in this book are even more relevant in the world of digital radiography because many digital radiography machines use more radiation than traditional film radiography. It is also too easy for technicians to repeat exposures and get sloppy with digital radiography. Some (irresponsible) digital radiography vendors even recommend "just repeating" exposures if there are image quality issues.

Good luck. Be Safe. Let us know if we can be of any help.
Matt Wright DVM MS DACVR

CHAPTER 1:

A (very) Short Guide to Radiation Safety for the Veterinary Technician

PART 1

BASIC RADIATION SAFETY

IN THIS PART:
- → Learn about the units of radiation
- → Know the ALARA concept
- → Know the acute and chronic effects of radiation injury
- → Know methods to decrease radiation exposure
- → Know the current recommended limits of radiation exposure
- → Understand the use of personnel radiation monitoring devices.

Remember the Incredible Hulk? Bruce Banner? Remember the gamma rays that turned him into a big green baby who got all bent out of shape when Bruce got upset and cried about something? In the real world that exposure to radiation, including gamma rays, will not turn you into a mutant. This is good news because as a veterinary technician you will be exposed to radiation for the rest of your career.

The questions all technicians ask is "how much radiation can I be exposed to and still be safe?" and "What are the real side effects?" The answers to those questions can be found in this chapter.

Before we can begin I must subject you to the mostest, boringest, worstest, 10 minutes of anything I have ever written and talk about the units of radiation. (This book really does get better after the first chapter. I promise.)

Units, units, units

You can't bake a cake if you don't know how much a cup of flour measures. Similarly, you can't talk about radiation safety if you don't know how much a "rad" of x-rays is. In this chapter, I talk about the units of radiation in "traditional units" and "SI units." The traditional units are used in America. The SI units are used everywhere else in the world and on the exposure badges you get back from some x-ray badge companies.

***Units of* Exposure**: This unit represents the amount of exposure you get. Think of it in terms of someone throwing jellybeans at you. If they throw 1000 jellybeans at you, you are exposed to 1000 jelly beans.

Roentgens measure the quantity of ionization of air produced by an x-ray or gamma ray. The unit is coulombs/kg of air.

***Units of* Absorbed Dose**: Simply, these units represent the amount of energy that is deposited within an absorber (your patient or your body). As far as the jellybean analogy goes, it is (kind of like) a measure of how many jelly beans will harm you and cause a welt and how many will just bounce off.

Rad: The traditional unit. It stands for the radiation-absorbed dose. The unit is ergs/gram.

Gray(Gy): The SI unit. Expressed in joules/kilogram.
Some useful conversions:
- 1 Gy=100 rad
- 1cgy=1rad
- 1rad=0.01Gy

***Units of* Dose Equivalents**: Simply, these units account for differences in tissue damage resulting from different types of radiation. Stated another way, these units allow you to compare the absorbed dose from two different kinds of radiation. Getting back to our jelly bean analogy, let's say someone is throwing jellybeans and rocks at you. The rocks will cause more damage. These units let you say something like "35 jelly beans create the same size bruise on my arm as 4 rocks."

In order to compare different types of radiation, each type of radiation is assigned a quality factor (QF). Radiations that cause more damage, such as neutrons, have a higher quality factor than those that cause less damage (like x-rays). The quality factor is multiplied by the absorbed dose to give you the dose equivalent.

Dose equivalent (rem or Sv) = absorbed dose (Gy or rad) x quality factor

Rem: The traditional unit. This stands for the roentgen equivalent man.

Sievert: the SI unit.
Some useful conversions:
- 1Sv=100rem
- 1rem=0.01Sv

These units are important because your exposure badge that you will wear any time you take radiographs is reported in Rem or Sv.

Ionization; the good, the bad, the ugly

Ionizing radiation is useful in medical diagnostics. Ionizing radiation, however, is also an environmental and occupational hazard.

You, the veterinarian or veterinary technician, are responsible for the radiation safety in your practice. You are responsible to register your x-ray machine with the appropriate state regulatory agency. (If you caught without a license it won't help to say that you didn't know you were supposed to have one. Be warned). You are responsible to assure that only properly trained personnel use any radiation source. You are also responsible to provide that training, enforcing the rules of radiation safety. So, for you to teach them, I must teach you. To begin...the ALARA concept.

ALARA: ALARA stands for **as low as reasonable achievable**. No concept could be any clearer. Keep exposure as low as reasonably achievable. This principle is based on the premise that all radiation exposure entails some degree of risk. All radiation is potentially harmful. Like acne when you are a teenager...the less - the better.

Radiation Injury: Keeping radiation exposure to an absolute minimum is important because radiation damages cells by disrupting the vital molecules in cells. The specific effects of radiation depend on a number of factors:

1. **The rate of delivery:** 650 rads administered in a single dose could kill a person. However, 650 rads administered over 50 years would be unlikely to result in detectable damage to anyone. One reason for this is that our bodies can repair tissues injured by radiation. This allows us to work with radiation and receive low levels each month and not show any untoward effects.
2. **The amount of the body exposed:** A high level of exposure can be tolerated if administered to a small portion of the body, while the same exposure would cause death if administered to the whole animal. We use this concept in radiation therapy where we administer high doses to small parts of an animal.
3. **The sensitivity of the individual and the variation of sensitivity of body cells**: Certain cells within the body are more radiosensitive than others. The most sensitive tissues are characterized by rapid division and lack of differentiation. Lymphocytes and all immature germ cells are highly sensitive to radiation injury. The cells lining the gastrointestinal tract are particularly sensitive. Other sensitive tissues include the thyroid gland, and the lens in the eye. Conversely, your arms and legs can withstand much higher doses of radiation than the

blood forming organs because of the decreased sensitivity of epithelial, muscle, and nerve tissue.

Ultimately, there are a number of factors that determine the body's response to radiation injury. Radiation injury may be acute and noted within days following whole body radiation; or it may be chronic and take years for the effect to manifest.

Acute effects: Acute effects are seen within a few days to weeks following whole body radiation. These effects include:
- Pancytopenia: Pancytopenia refers to the ablation of red cells and white cells. This results in hemorrhage and infection.
- Vomiting, diarrhea, dehydration due to death and sloughing of the intestinal lining cells.
- Neurological symptoms resulting from cerebral edema, vasculitis and meningitis. A much higher dose is required to cause neurologic problems than bone marrow and GI injury).

Keep in mind that these acute effects are not associated with diagnostic radiology. They may by seen with radiation therapy administered to treat some tumors. For the most part, acute effects are generally associated with atomic bombs and nuclear meltdowns. If you see these acute effects at your practice something is seriously wrong.

Chronic effects: Chronic effects may be seen months to years after radiation exposure. These are the effects you hear about in the news. Unfortunately, less is known about harmful effects from chronic exposure to radiation. The possible effects of radiation include:
- Genetic effects such as radiation induced mutation
- Increased risk of cancer with a higher incidence of skin tumors, thyroid tumors, and leukemia
- Increased fetal abnormalities with in utero irradiation such as growth retardation, congenital malformation, embryonic or fetal death, childhood leukemia.
  - Shortened life span with premature aging

- Cataract formation

The bottom line of all this radiation damage business is that radiation will cause damage. The less radiation you are exposed to the better. This is not meant to scare you or prevent you from performing your job.

Rather, it is meant to alert you to the potential hazards and scare you into following good radiation safety and protection procedures. If you follow prudent radiation safety practices you will have a safe and fulfilling career as an employee who works with radiation on a daily basis.

Time, Distance, Shielding

Follow of these three rules and you will decrease your exposure to radiation.

Rule #1 – **Reduce Exposure Time**: Reduce the amount of time your exposed to radiation and you reduce your exposure. Methods to reduce exposure time include:

- Use good radiographic techniques to avoid retakes. This includes always using a technique chart, taking time to position animals correctly, and use good film processing technique. If you avoid taking crummy films in the first place, you will have fewer retakes.
- If you are still using film radiography, use fast film and screens. Like we said before fast film means fewer x-rays are needed to expose the film.
- If you are using digital radiography – do not be sloppy. Just because it is easy and less expensive to repeat a projection does not mean you should do it in all cases. Do what you can to ensure proper positioning the first time.
- Remove all extraneous personnel from the area and position them at as great a distance from the source of the radiation as is practical. That means get all owners and people not intimately associated with holding the animal or operating the

radiographic equipment out of the examination area. Using sedation, sandbags, and tape to restrain patients so nobody is in the room during radiography is ideal.

Rule #2 – Maximize distance from the radiation source: This one is big, pay attention! There is a law of physics called the *inverse square law* which states that the reduction in radiation exposure decreases exponentially (squared) as you move farther and farther away from radiation source.

For example, if you double your distance away from a radiation source you decrease your exposure by a factor of four. Therefore, even if you can move just a little farther away from the x-ray tube you decrease your dose by a large amount. To put this law into practice:

- Stand as far away from the x-ray tube as possible when making in exposure. Also, minimize manual restraint by sedating animals or using positioning devices.
- Never hand-hold portable units. Always use portable stands
- Use cassette holders, do not hand hold cassettes
- If you must hold a patient, extend your arms and move your head and trunk away from the primary beam and source of radiation.
- Avoid manual restraint by sedating animals and using positioning devices.

Rule #3 – Use shielding: This rule basically states that if you can prevent the radiation from hitting you, you will get less exposure.

- Use beam-limiting devices and collimate to the appropriate field size.
- Use personnel protective shielding: keep in mind, **lead apron and gloves protect only against scatter radiation NOT the primary beam**. In other words, if your hand is in the radiograph *even if you are wearing a lead glove* your hand is not protected from the primary beam. This is why radiologists go off the wall when we see the outline of lead gloves in radiographs. When taking a radiograph you should wear:
  - A full body lead apron

- Protective gloves
- A thyroid shield

Protective eye glasses are also recommended. If you don't wear protective glasses, at least don't look at the x-ray tube during an exposure and avert your eyes from the patient.

The proper use of lead apron's and gloves is essential for radiation protection. Aprons and gloves should be checked periodically for cracks and defects. The apron should be hung and not folded. Folding causes cracks to form in the lead. In order to test for any cracks in the lead, simply radiograph your equipment. Cracks will show up as black areas on the film.

How much is too much?

So exactly how much radiation can you be exposed to and guarantee that you will not have any untoward effects? The answer of course is zero. Any radiation is harmful.

Unfortunately, there is no possible way you can be exposed to zero radiation. Attempting zero radiation exposure is simply not a realistic or practical goal expecially if you want to work in a veterinary practice.

The fact of the matter is that we live in a radiation field all of our lives. The radiation we are exposed to every day is referred to as "background radiation." We will talk more about this in a minute.

If trying to get zero exposure is impractical, the question remains, how much is O.K? To answer this question, The National Council on Radiation Protection (NCRP) developed the concept of *permissible exposure to* guide radiation workers toward acceptable limits.

The NCRP makes the following recommendations based on current knowledge (note these recommendations have become stricter over time as we learned more about the adverse effects of radiation and may change in the future):

- The **Maximum Permissible Dose** (MPD) is the dose above normal background radiation

- The MPD will depend on whether the person is classified as an occupational worker or as the general public.
- The minimum age of an occupational worker is **18 years old**. That means high school kids are not allowed to volunteer to take radiographs at your practice no matter how much they want to help.
- The limits of greatest concern to those working with diagnostic radiology relate to whole body dose which means exposure to any major portion of the whole body, head and trunk, gonads, lens of the eye, active blood informing organs, or the whole body.
- And the present time of the maximum whole body dose equivalents are:
  - For occupational workers = 5 rems/year (50msv)(5000mrem)
  - For the general public = 0.1 rem/year(1mSv)
  - For an embryo or fetus = 0.5rem/9months (5mSv) with 0.05 rem in any given month. Therefore, you should not allow pregnant women to obtain radiographs in your practice. You never know when they will require radiographs for their own medical purposes. (If they do, the baby must be badged (by wearing an additional badge under the apron at belly (baby) level).
- The maximum accumulated whole body does equivalent (lifetime dose) for occupational workers is 5(n-18) where "n" is in the age in years.

Putting things in Perspective – What do these doses mean to me?
(This is important – don't skim this part).
So far you have seen a lot of numbers but it is probably hard to understand what these numbers mean. A good way for some people to get a grasp of how much a millirem is to take a look at how much radiation exposure you get in some daily activities. Here you go:

- Getting out of bed eating food and being alive = 360mRem/

year. This is mostly from the food you eat, the rocks used to build the house you live in and the radon gas in your basement.
- 5 hour jet plane ride = 3mRem/5 hours (airline workers are classified as radiation workers in some countries!)
- Chest x-ray=8mrem
- Mammogram 138mRem
- CT scan = 2500mRem
- Smoking 20 cigarettes per day = 5300mRem to a smokers lung
- Cancer treatment = 5,000,000 mRem to the lung

Most of us probably won't get a CT scan or smoke 20 Marlboro's per day but, as you can see, you will get 360 mrem just from eating food and standing next to a rock. If you live in Denver or work as a lifeguard at a beach in the Caribbean your dose will likely be higher.

To give you some indication of the levels of radiation you will be exposed to if you follow good radiation safety protocols consider this: Recent studies have shown a low radiation exposure to veterinarians. The results determined for radiation detection devices distributed to a randomly selected sample of 118 women veterinarians showed that only 14.4 percent had documented exposures greater than 15mrem/month during the monitoring period measured under a lead apron. The maximally recorded whole body dose for one veterinarian was 44.2 mrem/quarter-year which was well below the maximum permissible dose of 1250 mrem/quarter year. *Patterns of ionizing radiation exposure among women veterinarians. J Am Vet Med Assoc. 1989 Sep 15;195(6):737-9.*

Keep in mind that even though the legal limit is 1250 mrem/qtr this is not acceptable in your practice. You should strive for at least ten times less than that. If your doses are higher you must figure out what is wrong and how you can improve the radiation safety in your practice.

With an understanding that 5000mrem is the MPD (maximum permissible dose) you can now have a meaningful discussion with your staff or with your employer about radiation safety. To begin this discussion you will need your quarterly radiation monitoring badge reading. Technicians should be given their badge reading and this number should be related to their MPD for the quarter/year/and lifetime cumulative dose.

I was recently working with a clinic where a technician saw her badge report and was terrified that she had an exposure of 28mRem for her lifetime dose. After our discussion, she understood that her MPD was 5000mrem/year so 28mrem was more than 100 times less than her exposure for a single year. Furthermore, her 28mrem was her lifetime occupational exposure. She had been working for three years. Therefore, her lifetime dose was 10,000 times less than her lifetime MPD of 5000 x 3=15,000! After our discussion, she understood that she was well below her MPD.

In most practices I evaluate, the exposure to technicians generally falls in the range of 10-20mrem per quarter. It is recommended that any technician receiving greater than 50mrem/quarter be counseled about radiation safety and safety practices enacted and enforced in the hospital to reduce the radiation exposure to the technical staff. If the technicians dose is persistently greater than 50-100 mrem/quarter, in the absence of a huge caseload, it is likely that they are not following proper radiation safety practices or possibly that they are mishandling their badge (leaving it in the x-ray room, on the dashboard of their car etc.) Speaking of badges...

Personnel Monitoring Devices (a.k.a Film Badges)

Personnel monitoring devices are used in long-term monitoring of low levels of radiation. Because our five senses cannot detect x-rays, some form of detector must be used to evaluate the radiation safety procedures that you are using. The most widely used personnel monitor is the nuclear emulsion monitor. It consists of a piece of film that is inserted in a special plastic holder which can be clipped your clothes. It is more commonly known as a *film badge*. Film badges are sent to a company to be read and report the results on a periodic basis. The length of time between evaluations depends on the amount of radiation to which the worker will be exposed. Quarterly readings are the most common in veterinary practice.

The film badge should be worn any time you are obtaining radiographs or are in the area of your hospital in which radiographs are obtained. The badge should be worn on the collar on the outside of the lead apron. This may seem inappropriate on first thought, however, the lens of the eye and the thyroid gland may not be protected from radiation under the lead apron. It is the exposure to these organs that becomes the critical exposure. It should be understood that the exposure to your body beneath the lead apron is much less than the reading on the film badge.

PART 2

RADIATION SAFETY FOR THE PREGNANT WORKER

IN THIS PART:
→ Learn about why radiation safety in the pregnant employee is a special situation
→ Learn about the Maximum Permissible Dose for the pregnant employee
→ Can a technician take radiographs during pregnancy?
→ Learn what an employee must do if they become pregnant?

Radiation Safety is Just Different for the Pregnant Employee

The fetus is particularly susceptible to the harmful effects of ionizing radiation during the first four months of pregnancy. Scientific studies have identified data that "are consistent with a lifetime cancer risk resulting from exposure during gestation which is two to three times that for the adult."

This special sensitivity must be considered when formulating a radiation safety protocol for the pregnant veterinary technician. The NRC states that the MPD for the pregnant patient is less than for other occupational workers. According to the NRC, the pregnant technician should not receive more than 500mrem of exposure during the entire pregnancy and less than 50mrem in any given month.

All pregnant employees should be given a copy of the United States Nuclear Regulatory Comission (NRC) Regulatory Guide 8.13 – Instruction Concerning Prenatal Radiation Exposure. The full text of this guide is included as Appendix 1 in this book and can be downloaded in electronic form at **http://www.stanford.edu/dept/ EHS/prod/researchlab/radlaser/regulatoryguide.pdf**

The million dollar question that is always asked by veterinarians and technicians is "can pregnant employees continue to take radiographs during pregnancy?"

This is a difficult question. Although state and local laws may vary (check with your state board), in many states and jurisdictions, technicians are able to continue obtain radiographs in a veterinary hospital if the hospital follows a strict protocol for radiation monitoring and safety during the pregnancy (see below). Nonetheless, a prudent and recommended approach (it is the approach I recommend and an approach that nobody will criticize) is to encourage technicians to stay out of the x-ray room for the duration of the pregnancy.

One of the important reasons we recommend keeping pregnant technicians out of the x-ray room is that the MPD for the pregnant worker is much lower than other radiation workers. You never know when a technician will require radiographs for their own medical purposes and you don't want to exceed their MPD during daily work just in case they need radiographs or a CT scan for health reasons during the pregnancy. It is my opinion, that this situation simply be avoided if at all possible.

If, for whatever reason, a technician insists on working in radiology during the pregnancy, or if working in radiology is an unavoidable requirement of employment, a strict radiation safety protocol that conforms to the NRC guidelines must be in place to protect the embryo-fetus from the harmful effects of ionizing radiation; and the veterinary hospital from liability if problems should arise related to the pregnancy. See Appendix 1 for more information.

Do this if you are pregnant or think you are pregnant

When a technician becomes pregnant they must alert their supervisor of the pregnancy and declare the pregnancy in writing. If the technician does not declare the pregnancy in writing, the technician's dose continues to be controlled under the normal dose limits for radiation workers.

In other words, in order for a pregnant worker to take advantage of the lower exposure limit and dose monitoring provisions, the woman must declare her pregnancy in writing to the employer. A form letter for declaring pregnancy is provided in Appendix 2 of this book or the licensee may use its own form letter for declaring pregnancy.

The declared pregnant worker (DPW) should then be counseled regarding their exposure history, safety aspects of the employee's work, the harmful effects of radiation exposure to the fetus, the proper radiation safety protocols used to protect the fetus, and provide the worker with an opportunity to ask questions. These items are outlines in the NRC regulatory guide and can be found in Appendix 1 of this book.

All DPW's should be given a copy of this document. A signed copy of this document should be kept on record.

If the technician elects to continue working in radiology, the technician is given two radiation monitoring badges. One badge is worn on the torso and the other badge worn over the abdomen. The badges must be submitted for evaluation on a monthly basis.

Exposures must be less than 50mrem per month during the pregnancy.

The monthly reports should be reviewed with the DPW and these reports should become part of the workers permanent dose history.

Contact your local or state radiation safety officer to make sure that you have taken all of the proper precautions.

The fetal dose limit will remain in effect until the DPW is known to no longer known to be pregnant, or informs their supervisor that they are withdrawing their declaration of pregnancy.

PART 3

CREATING A VETERINARY RADIOGRAPHIC TECHNIQUE CHART

IN THIS PART:
→ Learn how to create a technique chart
→ See an example of a completed technique chart

A technique chart is the backbone of any veterinary radiology department. Without one, you are destined to take crummy radiographs or radiate yourself or your staff with unnecessary retakes.

Fortunately, creating a technique chart is easy. Follow these 6 steps and you will be on your way.

Remember, you will need a different technique chart for each of the different studies you perform. That means you will need at least four different technique charts (thorax, abdomen, extremity, spine). You will need to understand a little physics to understand this guide. If you need a refresher I suggest you read my lecture series on the physics of diagnostic radiology found at **www.breedfreak.com**

You need a technique chart for most digital radiography systems. However, the rules for creating a technique chart for a digital radiography system are different than for film. If you are using a digital radiography system in your practice, you must consult your vendor for directions on how to create a technique chart for your particular system. The good old laws of physics do not apply to many digital radiographic systems. In digital radiography, image processing is very important and the image processing varies so much between systems that it is difficult to recommend general guides for creating a digital radiographic technique chart. If you have digital radiography in your practice, skip this chapter.

STEP 1 – Get your radiology house in order: A little preparation will make all the difference:

Have your processor serviced: This will ensure that development is accurate. Remember 90% of all processing errors happen in the dark room!

Be sure that you are using screens that are all the same age, speed, and manufacturer: Intensifying screens are not like a wardrobe... you cannot mix and match them. Every technique chart will be specific to the particular film screen combination you are using.

To create the technique chart use a dog that weighs about 40 pounds but is not overweight. It would be easiest if the dog is anesthetized.

STEP 2 – Select your mAs: In veterinary medicine patient motion is a great concern so we like to use a high mAs and low kVp technique. This allows us to increase contrast (because of the low kV) and increase speed (because of the high mAs).

The following are recommended mAs based on a rare earth speed intensifying screen[****]
- **Table top (no grid) extremity: 1.6mAs**
- **Thorax: 1.6mAs**
- **Abdomen: 5.0mAs**
- **Spine: 5.0mAs**

To set your machine for the mAs listed above remember you must set the mA and the time separately.

If your x-ray machine only has one mA station you just select your mA and pick the speed to give you the desired mAs. For example, if you have a 200mA station and you wanted to use 1.6mAs for a thoracic technique chart you would pick

- 200mA x 1/120sec = 1.6mAs (extremity)
- 200mA x 1/120sec = 1.6mAs (thorax)
- 200mA x 1/60sec = 5.0mAs (abdomen)
- 200mA x 1/30sec = 10mAs (spine)

If your x-ray machine has two mA stations I suggest that for extremity techniques you use the smaller of the mA stations (usually 100mA) and for all other applications you use the larger mA station (usually 300mA). In this case your settings would be as follows:

- 100mA x 1/60sec = 1.6mAs (extremity)
- 100mA x 1/60sec = 1.6mAs (thorax)
- 300mA x 1/60sec = 5.0mAs (abdomen)
- 300mA x 1/30sec = 10mAs (spine)

STEP 3 – Select your initial kVp: The next step is to create a "perfect" radiograph. To do that, we need to find a kVp to go along with our suggested mAs setting. To pick a starting kVp use Sante's Rule:

- **kVp=(2 x tissue thickness) + FFD + grid factor**

FFD is the film focus distance and is usually set to 40 inches in veterinary medicine.

The grid factor is how much extra kVp you will need to account for the grid you are using. Remember, grids increase contrast but require more radiation to achieve the same exposure. If you are using a...

- **5:1 grid add 6-8kVp**
- **8:1 grid add 8-10kVp**
- **12:1 grid add 10-15kVp**

Most traditional film veterinary applications use an 8:1 grid. If you know you are using a grid but don't know what kind of grid is under your table assume it is an 8:1 grid. With digital radiography the grid type may vary considerable or even be removed. Some digital radiography machines remove the effects of scatter with advanced image processing techniques rather than a grid.

Remember, grids are not used in table top techniques. If you are making a technique chart for a table top study, use 0 (zero) for the grid factor.

To demonstrate Sante's rule lets say you have a dog that measures 15cm thick at the widest point in the abdomen, an FFD of 40 inches, and you are using an 8:1 grid.. you would use 80kVp ((2 x 15) + 40 + 10).

STEP 4 – Expose the Perfect Film: The goal in this step is to obtain a radiograph with a "perfect" exposure. The technique you use to generate this radiograph will be used to create the rest of the technique chart. Therefore, take your time and make this radiograph as good as it can be. It may take 5 or 6 tries to get it right but the time you spend on this step will be worth it in the end.

To get started take a radiograph with the mAs I recommend above for each particular study and set your kVp according to Sante's rule. For example....if I were creating an abdominal technique, using a 40 inch FFD, an 8:1 grid, and my dog measures 15cm then I would expose a radiograph at 7.5mAs and 80kVp. Hopefully, that exposure will be in the ballpark and the radiograph will be fairly well exposed. Unfortunately this is not always the case...

...if the radiograph is too dark then decrease the kVp by 15%

...if the radiograph is too light then increase the kVp by 15%

After you use the 15% rule to get you closer, keep increasing or decreasing the kVp in small increments (5% or as needed) until you get the exposure just right.

STEP 5 – Make the Technique Chart: Now that you have a properly exposed radiograph, you are over the hump and the rest is easy. To create the technique chart simply start with your "perfect exposure" and interpolate to find the values of kVp for other measurements according to the following rules:

- **Subtract 2 kVp from the original kVp for each cm decrease from the original measurement.**
- **Add 2 kVp to the original kVp for each cm increase from the original measurement up to 80 kVp.**

- Add 3 kVp for each cm increase that places the kVp above 80 up to 100.
- Add 4 kVp for each cm increase that places the kVp above 100.

For example...let's say that we started with a perfect exposure of 7.5mAs at 80kVp and our patient measured 15cm we would make an abdominal technique chart as follows:

....

STEP 6 – Create a technique chart for each different study such as abdomen, thorax, extremity, spine. Repeat the above process to create these additional technique charts.

An Example Technique Chart

On the following pages there is an example of a technique chart I made for a local veterinary hospital. It will give you an idea of what a finalized technique chart should look like. Do not try to use this technique chart in your hospital. That would be about as good as useless.

DOG & CAT EXTREMITY (TABLE TOP)
100MA X 1/40 SEC = 2.5MAS

cm	kVp
2	48
3	50
4	52
5	54
6	56
7	58
8	60
9	62
10	64
11	66
12	68
13	70
14	72
15	74

DOG THORAX (BUCKY)
300MA X 1/60SEC = 5MAS

cm	kVp
8	56
9	58
10	60
11	62
12	64
13	66
14	68
15	70
16	72
17	74
18	76
19	78
20	80
21	83
22	86
23	89
24	92
25	95

CAT THORAX (TABLE TOP)
300MA X 1/60SEC = 5MAS
THORAX

cm	kVp
4	41
5	43
6	45
7	47
8	49
9	51
10	53
11	55

**If cat is thicker than 11cm treat as a small dog and use a bucky technique for dog thorax
**Also use this chart for cat whole body with emphasis on thorax

DOG ABDOMEN (BUCKY)
300MA X 1/40SEC = 7.5MAS

cm	kVp
8	56
9	58
10	60
11	62
12	64
13	66
14	68
15	70
16	72
17	74
18	76
19	78
20	80
21	83
22	86
23	89

CAT ABDOMEN (TABLE TOP)
300MA X 1/40SEC = 7.5MAS
THORAX

cm	kVp
4	34
5	36
6	38
7	40
8	42
9	44
10	46
11	48

**If cat is thicker than 11cm treat as a small dog and use a bucky technique for dog abdomen
**Also use this chart for cat whole body with emphasis on abdomen

DOG PELVIS/SPINE (BUCKY)
300MA X 1/30SEC = 10MAS
THORAX

cm	kVp
8	56
9	58
10	60
11	62
12	64
13	66
14	68
15	70
16	72
17	74
18	76
19	78
20	80
21	83
22	86
23	89
24	92
25	95

PART 4

SPECIAL CONSIDERATIONS FOR DIGITAL RADIOGRAPHY

IN THIS PART:
→ Learn about why more exposure results in better images with digital radiography
→ Understand the concept of "dose creep" and what you can do to avoid it

---

In some ways digital radiography is similar to film radiography. In other ways, it is very different. One way it differs is it's response to exposure. When the radiographic exposure used to obtain traditional film is changed, the image gets dark or light and there is a loss of contrast. With digital radiography, the contrast is maintained and (for the most part) images don't get dark or light. Rather, they get more or less noisy.

With digital radiography, there is a trade off between exposure and noise. Exposure is not related to the lightness or darkness of an image.

Noise Defined: Noise is defined as a "random variation in image brightness." Practically speaking, noise is the graininess, mottling, or textured appearance that is present in all medical images.

Although noise can give an image an objectionable appearance some noise is acceptable in digital radiographic images. The most important problem with noise is that noise can reduce the visibility of low contrast objects because the visibility threshold of low-contrast objects, is very noise dependent.

Exposure and noise with traditional film-screen radiography: With traditional film-screen radiography overexposing an image makes the images too dark with a loss of contrast and underexposing an image makes the image too light with a loss of contrast. Changing technique does nothing to alter the amount of noise or mottle in an image. The amount of noise is set by the film screen combination you are using. Since the individual film grains and phosphor crystals in the screens are very small we don't generally appreciate grainy film images unless a very fast (sensitive) film screen system is used.

Exposure and noise in digital radiography: If a digital radiographic detector (CR, Flat Panel or CCD) is improperly exposed the image does not get too light or too dark. The wide dynamic range of digital radiography maintains contrast and image appearance over a wide range of exposures. Rather, if you underexpose a digital radiographic system, a principal change to the images is that the image will get noisy. The following is an image of an unacceptably noisy and underexposed DR image:

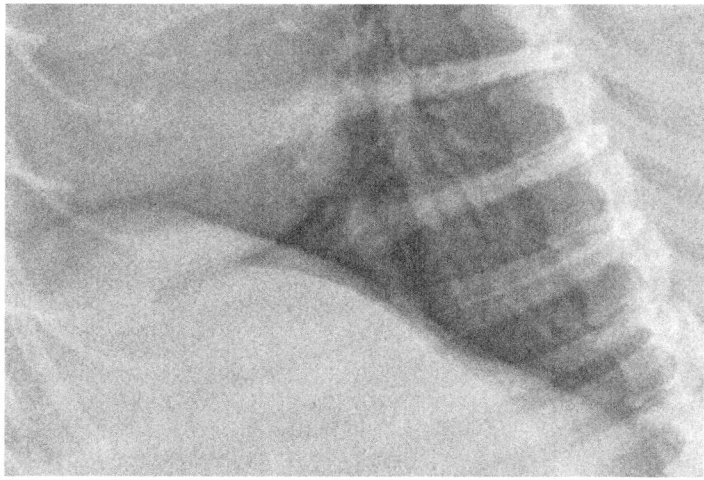

As you can see in the preceding image, the image does not get underexposed in the way that film gets underexposed. The primary change is that the image is more grainy. Just so you can see that the amount of noise will change with exposure, the following is an image taken with the exact same digital unit but the mAs was increased.

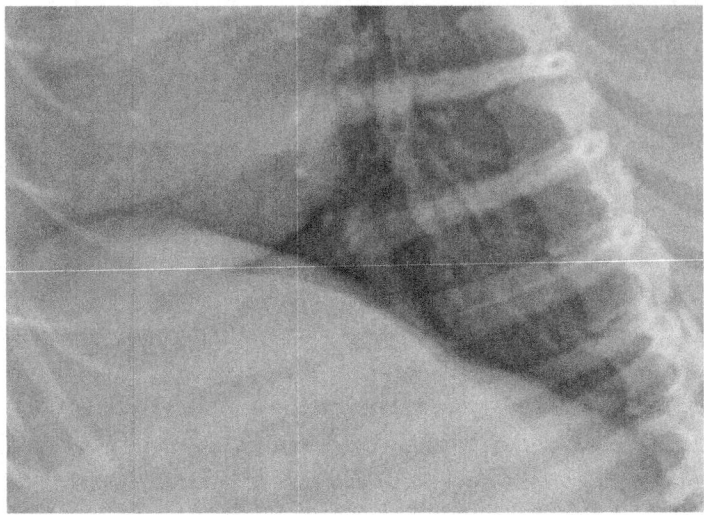

As you can see, there image is still properly exposed and diagnostic but there is still some noise in the image.

The presence of noise in an image is a trade off between exposure and the amount of noise in the image. With most digital detectors, if the technician cranks the exposure up enough the noise go away***.

Increasing the technique just to decrease noise is not recommended. A little noise is acceptable in digital radiographic images and increasing the technique simply to reduce noise will simply serve to unnecessarily expose patients and technicians. Overexposing patients in an effort to make a prettier image has been termed "dose creep."

As a general rule, CR (computed radiography) has less noisy images than DR (direct digital radiograpy) systems. Within the

DR category, the CCD (charge couple device) systems currently on the veterinary market appear to be more noisy than flat panel detectors but there is a huge variability between vendors as other factors such as image processing, scintillator type, number of pixels, CCD camera technology, electronic noise, crystal size (CR), CR phosphor packing density etc. impact the final image.

Veterinarians researching digital systems are often unaware of image noise and react (often violently) to the presence of noise in an image. Veterinarians must understand that digital images look different than film images and purchasing a digital system simply because the images "look like film images" can be limiting. Digital images look different than film and that takes some getting used to.

Some vendors smooth out their images so they don't appear noisy. This helps make sales as veterinarians (in my experience) who are new to digital radiography invariably will select a blurry image over a sharp grainy image. Unfortunately, this type of processing not only blurs the noise, but it blurs the anatomy depicted on the image as well. In our teleradiology practice, we consider blurry images much more objectionable than slightly noisy images because it can limit our ability to make a diagnosis.

Ways to decrease noise and prevent dose creep:

Technicians quickly learn that they get less complaints from veterinarians about their images if the images are not noisy. As stated previously, increasing technique just to decrease noise is not safe for them or for the patients. Technicians should be advised to try to prevent "dose creep."

1. A technique chart is recommended. This technique chart can be programmed into the anatomic programming of newer x-ray machines. Despite what the vendors say, the vast majority of the digital radiography systems need a technique chart. Do not accept a "generic" technique chart from your vendor. A

technique chart must be developed for your system on the day of the install.
2. Consideration should be given to purchasing a digital radiography system that provides technicians with an EXPOSURE INDEX. The exposure index tells the technicians if the image is properly exposed. Some digital radiography systems on the veterinary market now offer an exposure index.

....

In conclusion, image noise is a factor in digital radiography and the amount of noise present in an image should be a consideration when purchasing a system. Some systems have more noise than others. Eliminating noise in digital radiographic images is possible (for many systems) but (for many systems) would require an unnecessary increase in dose to the patient and personnel.

*** *Unfortunately, there are some detectors on the veterinary market that are so insensitive to radiation that the images are objectionably noisy regardless of technique. In my experience, these detectors are usually low end or older model CCD units.*

PART 5

COMMON SEDATION PROTOCOLS FOR VETERINARY RADIOGRAPHY

IN THIS PART:
→ Learn about common Sedation Protocols for Veterinary Radiography

---

Many dogs will allow themselves to be positioned for radiography using sandbags, rope, and tape without sedation. However, in many cases, sedation is required to position dogs without using manual restraint.

The following sedative protocols have been used to successfully position veterinary patients for radiography. It cannot be overstated that every sedative protocol carries some degree of risk to the patient and every patient receiving sedative medications must have a complete pre-sedative examination to help ensure that the patient is healthy enough to handle the procedure. All sedation must be administered by a veterinarian or under the supervision of a licensed veterinarian.

YOUNG DOGS	Buprenorphine 0.01mg/kg IV Acepromazine 0.05mg/kg IV Atropine 0.02mg/kg IV
OLDER DOGS	Butorphanol 0.1-0.4mg/kg IV Diazepam 0.2-0.5mg/kg IV
FRACTIOUS CATS	Midazolam 0.2cc IM Ketamine 0.2cc IM Butorphanol 0.2cc IM
"REGULAR CATS"	Midazolam 0.1cc IV Ketamine 0.1cc IV Butorphanol 0.1cc IV

PART 6

TWO CHARTS TO PRINT OUT AND POST ON THE WALL

IN THIS PART:
→ The 4 Pillars of Veterinary Radiation Safety
→ Evaluating the improperly exposed radiograph

The following pages are essentially a summary of what we have already discussed and a "cheat sheet" for technicians to use if they run into problems in the x-ray room. Many practices have charts with this (or similar) information printed on the wall in the x-ray room.

THE FOUR PILLARS OF VETERINARY RADIATION SAFETY

Time:
- Minimizing time exposed to ionizing radiation is advised
- Use technique charts to decrease repeat examinations
- Rotate available personnel so no worker spends a disproportionate amount of time producing radiographs
- Use tape, sandbags, sedation, and restraint devices to limit manual positioning of animals
- Plan the radiographic procedure carefully in order to avoid repeat films
- Use film screen systems that minimize the time of exposure

Distance:
- Maximize the distance between the worker and the x-ray beam
  - **Remember**: The radiation exposure is inversely proportional to the distance from the x-ray machine. In other words, small increases in distance result in large decreases in exposure.
- Remove all essential personnel from the radiology room during exposure
- Never hand hold a cassette – even with a gloved hand

*The rules are recommended radiation safety practices that will minimize exposure to ionizing radiation. All workers should be advised that all radiation is potentially harmful. The NCRP is a government advisory group that recommends radiation safety practices for health care workers. The NCRP Report No. 36 pertains to the use of diagnostic x-ray's in veterinary medicine. The use of diagnostic radiation in most veterinary practices is regulated by state or local governments.

Shielding:

- Always wear protective aprons
- Always wear protective gloves
- Always wear a thyroid shield
- Never allow any pert of the workers body to be in the primary beam:
  - **Remember**: Lead only protects you from scatter radiation
  - **Remember**: Lead aprons and gloves do not protect you from the primary beam

Common Sense:

- Avoid the primary beam
- Never hold a portable x-ray machine during the exposure
- Do not allow pregnant women or personnel younger than 18 years old in the radiology room
- To reduce scatter collimate around your patient so there is a 1-inch unexposed area at the periphery of your radiograph in all studies
- Wear a film badge outside your lead apron at neck level to monitor radiation dose
- Look away during exposures to protect the lens of the eye

EVALUATING THE IMPROPERLY EXPOSED RADIOGRAPH

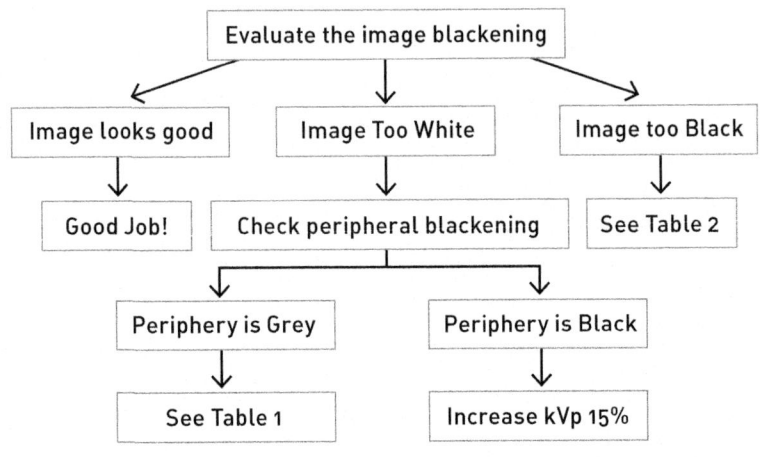

TABLE 1: FILM IS TOO LIGHT	TABLE 2: FILM IS TOO BLACK
Common Causes Insufficient Technique: • Increase mAs by 50% • Increase kVp by 15% Used the Wrong Technique Chart X-ray tube not aligned with Grid X-ray tube height is too high Measured Incorrectly	**Common Causes** Excessive Technique Decrease mAs by 50% Decrease kVp by 15% Double Exposure X-ray tube height is too low
Less Common Causes: Processor Problems Developer Exhausted Developer diluted Inadequate Developer Replenishment Developer Temperature too low Processor Timer Malfunction	**Less Common Causes:** Processor Problems Developer too strong Developer temperature too high Processor timer malfunction
	Less Common Causes: Darkroom Problems Light Fog Safety Light Malfunction
Rare Causes X-ray machine miscalibration X-ray tube failure X-ray machine timer malfunction	**Rare Causes** X-ray machine timer malfunction X-ray machine miscalibration

Radiograph quality evaluation for exposure variables – a review. Vet Radiol Ultrasound. 1999 May-Jun;40(3):220-6.)

PART 7

EQUIPMENT YOU WILL NEED TO NON-MANUALLY RESTRAIN YOUR PATIENTS

IN THIS PART:
→ Learn about the equipment necessary to restrain patients with sandbags and tape

Fortunately, there are very few pieces of equipment that you will need to perform non-manual restraint in your veterinary practice. Sandbags, foam positioners, muzzles, mama clamps, tape, rope, and a method of affixing your ropes to the x-ray table are all that are necessary.

Sandbags: Sandbags may be the most important item used in non-manual restraint for veterinary radiography. Rule #1: don't buy cheap sandbags. They will spring leaks in no time and you will have sand all over your radiology room.

Sandbags can also be home made. If you are going to make them yourself be sure to make them very sturdy. Nothing is worse than having one break open in the middle of a busy day and have sand sprayed around the radiology suite.

Some technologists fill their sandbags with #7 buckshot. Using buckshot will make the bag act more like a large bean bag and may be more moldable. We are told that if a buckshot sandbag does happen to break open, you can clean the buckshot up with a large magnet.

Foam positioners: non-opaque foam positioners are highly recommended. Be careful and don't spill barium on them.

Muzzles: A good set of muzzles will come in handy. We routinely muzzle of our patients if they are not sedated. The muzzle seems to have a calming effect and gives the pet something to think about. You must get a good set of muzzles in a variety of sized for best effect. Pugs and Chows require special shaped muzzles.

Tape: Any kind of tape will do here. Most vets have white porous white tape on hand. Be careful not to tape limbs too tightly. It is easy to cut off circulation with tape.

Super Scruffers: These are nontraumatic clamps used to help restrain cats by "scruffing" them.

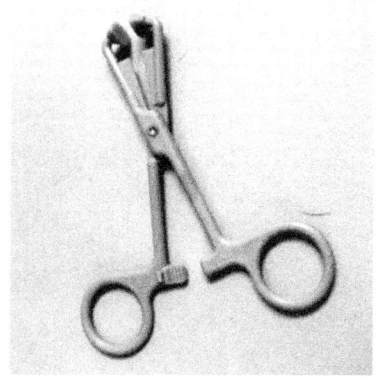

Super Scruffers can be purchased through your veterinary distributor.

Rope: having some good solid rope handy will help. We use ropes from an outdoor supply store (such as REI) that are used for rock climbing. Animals may elect to chew on these ropes so they must be sturdy.

Loc-A-Leg or other method of affixing rope to the x-ray table: in several of the images used in this book, you will notice this restraining device attached to the end of our x-ray table such as seen in the following images:

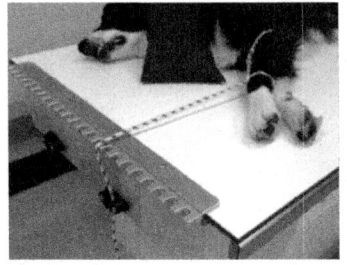 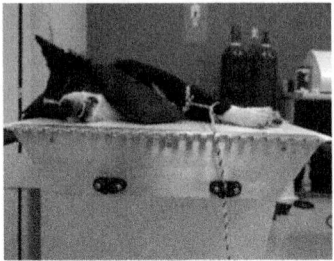

This device was developed exclusively for the veterinary market and is available at https://loc-a-leg.com/Home_Page.php

....

Pawsitioner: The Pawsitioner is a novel restraint device that is new on the veterinary market. This is an "all in one" restraint device that can be used to position dogs and cats in lateral and ventral dorsal recumbency for non-manual patient restraint during radiography.

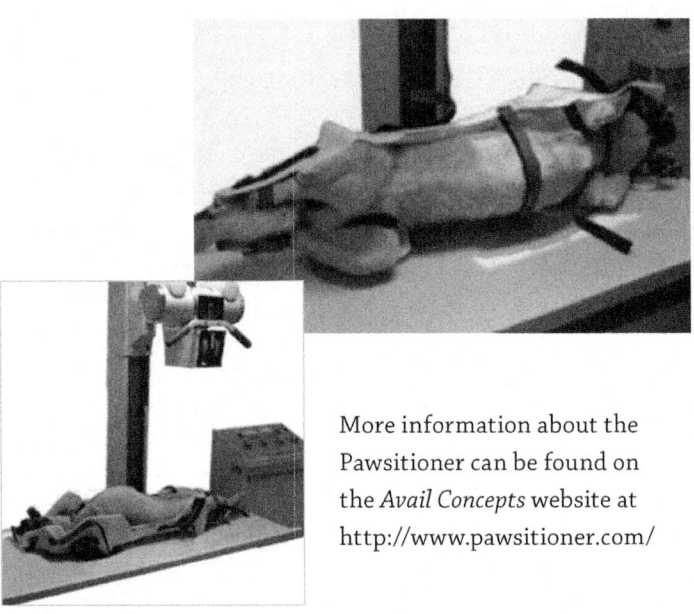

More information about the Pawsitioner can be found on the *Avail Concepts* website at http://www.pawsitioner.com/

PART 8

TECHNICAL BASICS OF POSITIONING PATIENTS FOR RADIOGRAPHY

IN THIS PART:
→ Learn our quick and dirty guide to positioning patients for radiography

Good radiographic technique will require a thorough knowledge about how to position patients as well as where to aim the radiographic beam. The following is a quick and dirty guide to get the most out of your time in the radiology room.

The primary goal of this book is to give technicians the basics of radiation safety and to teach them how to position patients using sandbags, rope, and tape. Therefore, a full discussion of all of the different radiographic projections is outside the scope of this text.

In this chapter we include some of our tips and tricks that we find useful. This will give you just enough background about the technical aspects of radiography to make you dangerous.

If you are unfamiliar with any of the projections described in this chapter, I highly suggest that you do some reading and get a good book that has pictures of all of the veterinary projections, positioning terminology, when the various projections are used, and where to collimate the light beam.

For further information about the technical aspects of radiography, I recommend the excellent "cook-book" for performing radiographs (including line drawings and radiographs of these projections) *Radiography in Veterinary Technology* by Lisa M. Lavin, C.V.T., A.A.S. (W. B. Saunders Company ISBN 0-7216-6686-8).

Abdominal Radiographs

Standard Projections
- The standard views are a lateral and ventral-dorsal projection. Always obtain 2 views for abdominal radiography

Landmarks
- Center on top of the last rib on canine abdominal radiographs (not behind it).
- Center two fingers behind last rib on all feline abdominal radiographs.
- If the animal's abdomen is longer than the film, choose a larger film or take additional caudal views
- Always take a lateral and VD projection. Note: If GDV suspect then be sure that you obtain a right lateral projection.
- These landmarks apply for both the lateral and ventral dorsal projection

Technique
- Measure where you center.
- Technique charts are based on an average animal. You will need to adjust your technique for animals that are particularly fat or thin.

Tips
- Palpate your landmarks. Don't guess where your landmarks are.
- Use a larger film than you think you need. Remember, animals elongate when positioned properly!
- Be sure to include the diaphragm and the cranial portion of the pelvis in all abdominal radiographs.
- Use an 11 X 14 size plate on feline abdominal radiographs. (Exception – kittens).

- Extend the rear limbs so they do not overlie the bladder or prostate.
- The light field should extend from the tip of the sternum to the base of the tail.
- Repeat films as necessary until the study is complete and properly exposed.
- DV radiographs of the abdomen are unacceptable. If necessary, sedate the animal to obtain properly positioned radiographs.
- Obtain the radiographs at end expiration as there will be less breathing motion.

Thoracic Radiographs

Standard Projections
Two projections are necessary. A right or left lateral; and a ventral dorsal or dorsal ventral projection are necessary.

Landmarks
- Always pull the front legs forward.
- **With the front legs pulled forward, center at the caudal aspect of the scapula in both the lateral and VD/DV projections. In larger dogs center the width of two fingers caudal to the scapula.**
- **Position the center of the x-ray beam on the caudal edge of the scapula in the lateral and ventral dorsal projections.**
  - If the animal's thorax seems to be bigger than the film, always chose a larger film. (The cost savings from using a smaller size film are negligible! The expense of repeating a radiograph because you chose film that is too small is high)
  - Be absolutely sure that the area included on your radiograph includes the entire thorax from the sternum to the lateral vertebral processes of the spine. *Do not worry about including the entire dorsal-spinous processes.* Remember, we are radiographing the thorax and not the backfat!

Technique
- Measure where you center with the animal in correct position (measure with the animal lying on the x-ray table).
- Technique charts are formulated for the average animal. You will have to adjust your technique for obese or thin animals as well as animals with pleural effusion or severe pulmonary disease.

Tips
- Palpate your landmarks! Don't guess where your landmarks are.
- Use a larger film than you think you need. Remember, animals elongate when positioned properly.
- Use a 10 X 12 on all cats for thoracic radiographs (*Exception – kittens*).
- Always pull the front legs forward so they are touching the nose of the animal. This will ensure that you move the triceps muscle mass away from the cranial thorax.
- Repeat films as necessary until the study is complete and properly exposed.
- Expose the radiograph on maximum inspiration.
- Collimator light field:
  - In the lateral projection, the collimator light field should start at the shoulder and end caudal to the last rib.
  - In the ventral dorsal projection, the collimator light field should run the length of the cassette and extend to the width of the thorax.
  - Always do both lateral projections if you are looking for metastatic disease.

A foam wedge placed under the sternum is necessary in most large breed dogs. Some of the smaller barrel-chested dogs may require the wedge sponge placed under the dorsal spinous processes. (Tip: palpate the sternum and the dorsal spinous processes. They should level and parallel to the table.)

Extremity Radiographs

Technical accuracy is essential to obtaining diagnostic extremity radiographs. In general, problems encountered with extremity radiography fall into two equally important categories. These are:

- **Exposure problems:** Overexposed (too dark) extremity radiographs are a very common problem in veterinary radiography. Many times, a lack of collimation around the bone in question is the cause of overexposed radiographs. To correct this problem you must be sure that you collimate closely around the bone in question. In a properly collimated radiograph, there should only be an inch of exposed film surrounding the extremity in question. Close collimation will reduce scatter and therefore prevent overexposed radiographs.
- **Positioning Problems:** A guide to positioning extremity radiographs is outside of the scope of this handout, however, if you are having problems obtaining properly positioned radiographs you should consider sedating the animal for radiography. The expense of sedation is far outweighed by the risk of missing a small lesion by trying to interpret obliqued radiographs. In fact, some radiologists say that you cannot consistently obtain properly positioned extremity radiographs without the benefit of sedation!

Landmarks
- **For joint integrity** – center on the joint.
- **For long bones or fractures** – center on the mid-shaft of the bone and be sure to include the joint above and below the bone in question within the collimated light field.

Technique
- Use a tabletop technique (no grid) if the extremity in question is less than 10cm thick. *When performing tabletop radiography, don't forget to change the tube height (raise the tube) to the tabletop position.*
- Measure where you center the x-ray beam, with the animal lying on the x-ray table.

- Technique charts are based on an average animal. You will need to adjust your technique for excessively well-muscled or frail animals.
- Reduce the MAS by half for really tiny animals and exotics.

Tips
- Palpate your landmarks. Don't guess where they are.
- Place the injured side down for lateral view.
- Position the whole body so that that extremity you are radiographing is straight.
- Collimate, collimate, collimate!!!
- Repeat films as necessary until the study is complete and properly exposed.
- Always separate out the different parts of the limb with different projections. Whole leg radiographs are difficult to position and interpret.

Spinal Radiographs

Introduction

If you have had difficulty obtaining spinal radiographs in the past you are not alone. Spinal radiography can be tricky. Fortunately, if you follow the following rules you will be well on your way to decreasing the stress you feel when asked to take spinal radiographs. The following rules are mandatory for success.

Rule #1: **Always use general anesthesia** (or at the least heavy chemical restraint). Anesthesia is necessary to relax the musculature supporting the spine. Without it you will be in the "no mans land" of trying to interpret oblique radiographs.

Rule #2: **Use radiolucent sponges to position all views.**

Rule #3: **All films should be collimated closely around the spine to reduce scatter.** Use a collimator opening as long as the size of film chosen and collimate side to side.

Rule #4: **Measure where you center the x-ray beam.** It should be noted that this is not necessarily at the highest point.

Rule #5: **Keep track of your technical factors.** This will be helpful if you need to repeat a film and/or if the veterinarian will be performing myelography.

Lateral Spine Radiographs
- The animal should be positioned in lateral recumbency with the mid-saggital plane parallel to the table. *This usually requires a wedge sponge under the nose, one sponge under the neck to support the sag of the spine (between shoulder and head), and a wedge under the sternum (if needed) to raise the sternum so that it is parallel with the dorsal spinous processes The necessity of using radiolucent sponges to properly position the spine cannot be overstated.*
- Ideally the rear limbs should be stretched caudally with tape or sandbags to reduce the kyphotic curve at the T-L junction.
- You will need five separate radiographic projections to image the entire spine.
- The following describes where you should center your x-ray beam:
  - **Cranial Cervical** – The central ray should be directed at ~ C3. To locate this site, palpate the wings of the atlas and center the x-ray beam the length of one vertebra caudal to the wings.
  - **Caudal Cervical** – The central ray should be directed at C7-T1. To locate this site, palpate the first dorsal spinous process (between the shoulder blades) and the manubrium (sternal notch). Then mentally draw a line between these two points and center at the center of this line. Generally, this is the center of the spine of the scapula.
  - **Thoracic Spine** – This film should include T1 and T13 (So choose an adequate size (i.e. long) cassette. Center halfway between T1 and T13. (The KV should be reduced by 10% from technique chart listing, for this film only, because there will be less x-ray interaction with the air in the lungs.)

- **Thoraco-Lumbar Junction** – This film is centered at T13 - L1. To locate this site, palpate where the last rib attaches to the spine at T13. If this cannot be palpated you might use a point centered over the spine but half way between the last rib and the xiphoid process.
- **Lumbar Spine** – This film should include T13 and S1 (so choose an adequate size [i.e. long] cassette). Center halfway between T13 and S1, generally about the length of 2 vertebrae cranial to the ilial wings of the pelvis.

Ventral-Dorsal Spinal Radiographs
- Position the animal in straight ventro-dorsal recumbency with the mid-saggital plane perpendicular to the table. To accomplish this, support the neck with a sponge located caudal to the occipital protuberance and one cranial to the shoulders. (This will drop the mandible parallel with the table.) Sandbags, tape, or sponges can be used to support the body in ventro-dorsal position.
- You will need five separate radiographic projections to image the entire spine.
- The following describes where you should center your x-ray beam:
  - **Cranial Cervical** – Palpate the wings of the atlas and center the length of one vertebra caudal to that site.
  - **Caudal Cervical** – Because you are no longer able to palpate the first dorsal spinous process, palpate the joint between the manubrium and the body of the sternum, and center there. You will usually be successful in locating C7-T1. (This is usually palpated as a dip or a ridge in the sternum just caudal to the sternal notch.)
  - **Thoracic Spine** – Again this film should include T1 and T13, so choose the appropriate size of cassette. This projection should be centered halfway between T1 (which you located in the previous projection) and T13 which you will learn to locate in the next step.

- **Thoraco-lumbar Junction** – T13-L1 can found by palpating the xiphoid process and the bend of the last rib (as you would center for an abdominal film). To locate T13, take these two points and center halfway between the two on the mid-saggital plane.
- **Lumbar Spine** – This film should include T13 and S1, so choose the appropriate size of cassette. Center halfway between T13 and S1, generally about the length of 2 vertebrae cranial to the ilial wings of the pelvis. The umbilicus is generally a successful centering site.

Skull Radiographs

Introduction

Obtaining quality skull radiographs need not be difficult if you remember the first rule of skull radiography. This rule is *that the only way to obtain good quality skull rads is to obtain them with the animal under general anesthesia.* The corollary to this rule is that you are wasting your time if you try to get skull radiographs on a non-anesthetized dog. In case you missed it the first two times, general anesthesia will allow you to properly position the animal. **Radiolucent sponges should be used in positioning for all views.**

There are at least half a dozen projections you could obtain when evaluating the skull. All of these views are not necessary in all cases. Rather, I recommend that you begin every skull series with a closed mouth ventro-dorsal projection and a lateral projection of the skull with the technique set for the cranial vault (i.e. measure at the widest portion of the cranial vault). This will allow you to evaluate the whole skull for fractures and bony erosion through the cribiform plate. Once you have those two projections, you should obtain other projections based on the patients clinical signs (i.e. tympanic bullae, sinuses, fractures, visible masses, and dental arcades.)

Mandatory Projections In All Skull Series:
- *Lateral Skull Projection:*
  The animal should be positioned in lateral recumbency with affected side down and the mid-saggital plane parallel to the table.
  - This usually requires a wedge sponge under the nose, one sponge under the neck to support the sag of the spine (between shoulder and head), and a wedge under the sternum (if needed) to raise the sternum so that it is parallel with the dorsal spinous processes.
  - Center in the center of the head as a whole. Direct the central ray halfway between the occipital protuberance and the rostral nose and half-way between ventral and dorsal.
  - Set your technique by measuring at that centering point.
  - It is essential that you position the dog properly for this lateral projection because positioning for the tympanic bullae, mandible, maxilla, and dental arcades should be initiated from straight lateral recumbency.

- *Ventro-Dorsal Skull Radiograph*
  - Position the animal in straight ventro-dorsal recumbency with the midsaggital plane perpendicular to the table.
  - Support the neck with a sponge located just caudal to the occipital protuberance and cranial to the shoulders. (This will drop the mandible parallel with the table.)
  - Sandbags, tape, or sponges can be used to support the body in ventrodorsal recumbency.
  - If you look at the rostral end of the animal, the intra-orbital line should be parallel to the table and the mid-saggital plane should be perpendicular to the table.
  - Center in the center of the head as a whole. Direct the central ray halfway between the occipital protuberance and the rostral nose and half-way between lateral sides. Set your technique by measuring at that centering point.

Additional Positions for Evaluating Select Areas of the Skull

Sinuses and nasal cavity:
- *Lateral projection to evaluate the nasal cavity*
  - Positioning for the lateral view of the sinuses is the same as for the lateral view of the skull with just two changes, technique and central ray location.
  - The animal should be positioned in lateral recumbency with affected side down and the mid-saggital plane parallel to the table.
  - This usually requires a wedge sponge under the nose, one sponge under the neck to support the sag of the spine (between shoulder and head), and a wedge under the sternum (if needed) to raise the sternum so that it is parallel with the dorsal spinous processes.
  - Center in the center of the sinus cavities. Direct the central ray half-way between the caudal portion of the frontal sinus and the rostral nose and half-way between the hard palate and the dorsal surface of the nose.
  - Set your technique by measuring at that centering point. Another option for setting technique is to reduce the mAs (time) by half from the original lateral view of the skull.

- *Open mouth ventro-dorsal projection to evaluate the nasal cavity*
  - Initiate positioning for this view from straight ventro-dorsal position.
  - Support the neck with a sponge under it, caudal to the occipital protuberance and cranial to the shoulders. (This will drop the mandible parallel with the table.)
  - Sandbags, tape, or sponges can be used to support the body in ventro-dorsal recumbency.
  - If you look at the rostral end of the animal, the intra-orbital line should be parallel to the table and the mid-saggital plane should be perpendicular to the table.
  - Use a length of tape to secure the maxilla (caudal to the canine teeth) parallel to the table.

- Use another length of tape to bring the tracheal tube, tongue, and mandible as close to perpendicular to the table as possible.
- Center in the center of the maxillary sinus. If you are not able to bring the mandible to perpendicular to the table a 15° caudal tube angle could be used.
- Measure at that centering point, set the technique and take the radiograph. Another option for setting technique would be to reduce the mAs (time) by half from the technique used for the original ventro-dorsal.

- *Dorso-ventral Intra Oral View to visualize the rostral nasal cavity*
  - Support the thorax in dorso-ventral recumbency with the midsaggital plane perpendicular to the table.
  - Support the mandible parallel to the table.
  - Insert the corner of the film into the mouth.
  - Direct the central ray to the mid point of the maxillary sinus. Measure the nasal cavity and set the technique accordingly for the type of film you are using.

- *Rostro-caudal projection to evaluate the frontal sinus*
  - Initiate positioning for this view from straight ventro-dorsal position.
  - Support the neck & head with a sponge under it.
  - Sandbags, tape, or sponges can be used to support the body in ventro-dorsal recumbency.
  - If you look at the rostral end of the animal, the intra-orbital line should be parallel to the table and the mid-saggital plane should be perpendicular to the table.
  - Use a length of tape across the bridge of the nose to elevate the mid-saggital plane to perpendicular from the table.
  - Direct the central ray at the center of the intra-orbital line right on the mid-saggital plane.
  - Measure from the intra-orbital line to the table to determine technique settings.

Tympanic Bulla
- *Open mouth rostro-caudal projection to evaluate the tympanic bulla*
  - Initiate positioning for this view from straight ventro-dorsal position.
  - Support the neck & head with a sponge under it.
  - Sandbags, tape, or sponges can be used to support the body in ventro-dorsal recumbency.
  - If you look at the rostral end of the animal, the intra-orbital line should be parallel to the table and the mid-saggital plane should be perpendicular to the table.
  - Wrap a length of tape around the mandible, tracheal tube, and tongue.
  - Use that tape to elevate the head so that the maxilla is perpendicular to the table leaving the mouth open and the mandible at an angle of approximately 45°.
  - Measure from the table-top to the open corner of the mouth to set your technique.

- *Oblique Projections of the Tympanic Bullae*
  - Position the animal in straight lateral recumbency with the side down that you intend to profile.
  - Positioning for straight lateral recumbency usually requires a wedge sponge under the nose, one sponge under the neck to support the sag of the spine (between shoulder and head), and a wedge under the sternum (if needed) to raise the sternum so that it is parallel with the dorsal spinous processes.
  - Tilt the mid-saggital plane of the head dorsally not more than 20°.
  - Center over the bulla just caudal to the ramus of the mandible.
  - Measure at that centering point, set the technique and take the radiograph. Another option for setting technique is to reduce the mAs (time) by half from the original lateral view of the skull.

- Roll the animal over and repeat steps 1-4 for the opposite oblique.

Mandible and Maxilla
- *General recommendations:* The animal should be positioned in lateral recumbency with affected side down and the mid-saggital plane parallel to the table. This usually requires a wedge sponge under the nose, one sponge under the neck to support the sag of the spine (between shoulder and head), and a wedge under the sternum (if needed) to raise the sternum so that it is parallel with the dorsal spinous processes.

- *Oblique projection of the dental arcades*
    - Use a mouth speculum or appropriate size needle cap (between maxillary and mandibular canine teeth on one side) to prop the mouth to the open position.
    - Looking straight down into the open mouth, rotate the head until you see the dental arcade or ramus with out any overlying structures. Prop the head in that position with radiolucent sponges.
    - Center in the center of the part you are radiographing from rostral to caudal.
    - Measure at that centering point, set the technique and take the radiograph. Another option for setting technique is to reduce the mAs (time) by half from the original lateral view of the skull.

- *Ventro-dorsal view of the rostral mandible*
    - This position originates with the animal in ventro-dorsal recumbency.
    - Support the neck & head with a sponge under it.
    - Sandbags, tape, or sponges can be used to support the body in ventro-dorsal recumbency.

- If you look at the rostral end of the animal, the intra-orbital line should be parallel to the table and the mid-saggital plane should be perpendicular to the table.
- Place the corner of the film into the mouth as far as you can. Support the free end of the film with sponges.
- Measure the mandible and set the technique accordingly.

CHAPTER 2

Positioning with Sandbags, Rope, and Tape

Now for the good stuff. The remainder of this book contains step by step pictures about how to position pets with sandbags, rope, and tape. In the real world, you will have to get creative with your restraint technique. Use these images as a guide but think outside of the box and come up with your own techniques.

To keep book publishing costs down, we did not repeat every single projection for the dog and cat and we did not include every possible projection. In practice, you will get the hang of things if you follow this guide for positioning in the projections that we show. Ultimately, you really only have to learn how to position a patient in a basic VD and lateral position and then position the extremities as needed for extremity projections.

Good luck. We are always available to help. If you are having problems with positioning, send us your images. We are always available to troubleshoot and give assistance. You can always reach us online at **www.animalinsides.com** or through our teleradiology service at **www.insightradiology.net**

You will find that many of the techniques are shown using a Loc-A-Leg restraining device (see page 41 or email **positioner@animalinsides.com** for more information) but we also included several images using only sandbags, rope, and tape if you don't have a method of affixing ropes to the table.

Lateral Thorax or Lateral Abdomen of the Dog

STEP 1:
Secure the front legs

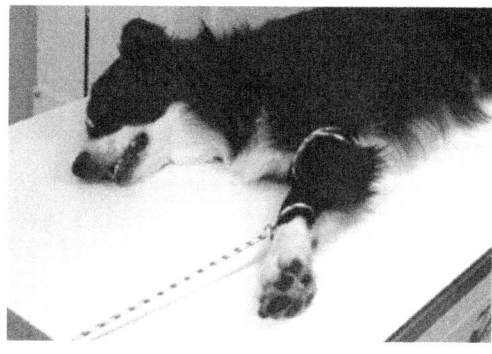

STEP 2:
Secure the back legs

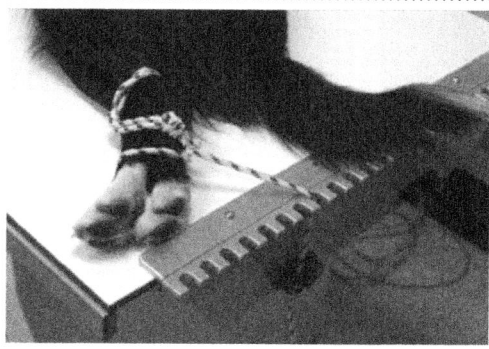

STEP 3:
Place a wedge under the sternum to elevate the sternum. Sandbags may be applied over the neck and pelvis if needed. This is how a fully restrained dog should be positioned.

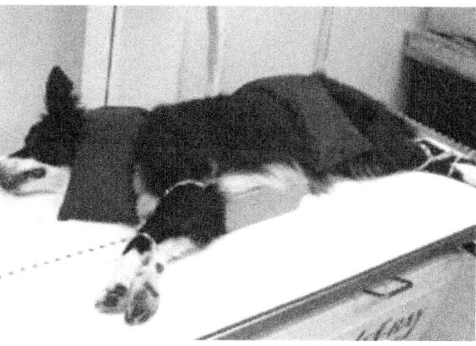

Lateral Thorax or Lateral Abdomen Cat

STEP 1:
Place non-traumatic forceps on cat scruff and secure the front legs to the table

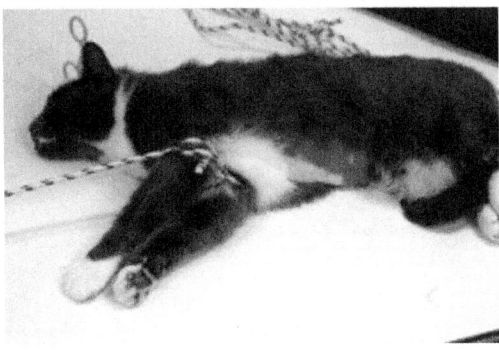

STEP 2:
Secure the hind legs to the table

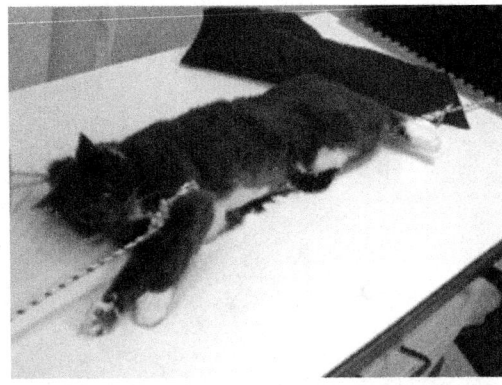

STEP 3:
This is what a properly positioned patient looks like

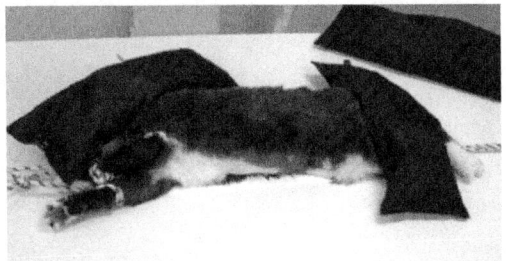

Ventral Dorsal Radiographs of the Thorax or Abdomen of the Cat

STEP 1:
Tape the back legs to the table

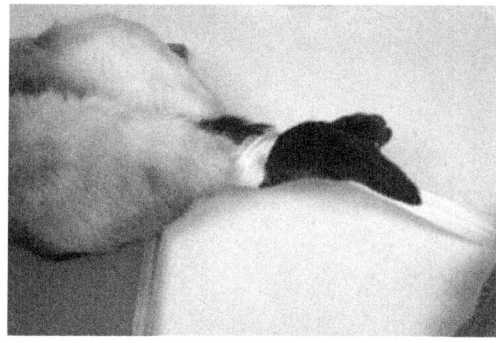

STEP 2:
Place a lead glove over the hind legs

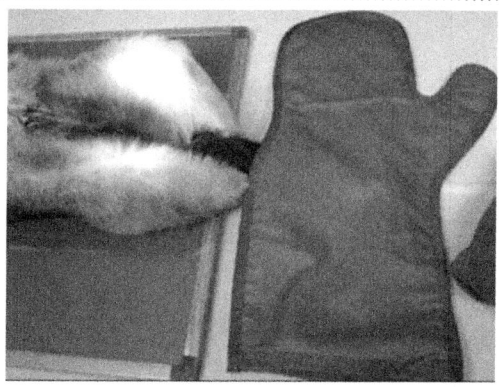

STEP 3:
Tape the front legs to the table

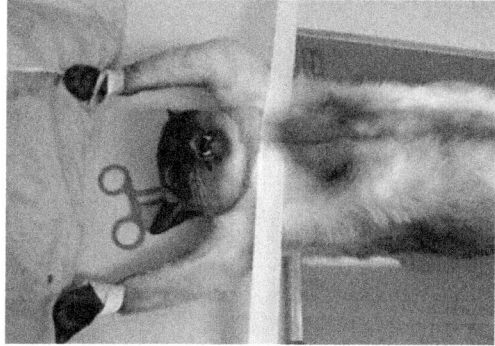

Ventral Dorsal Radiographs of the Thorax or Abdomen of the Cat - CONTINUED

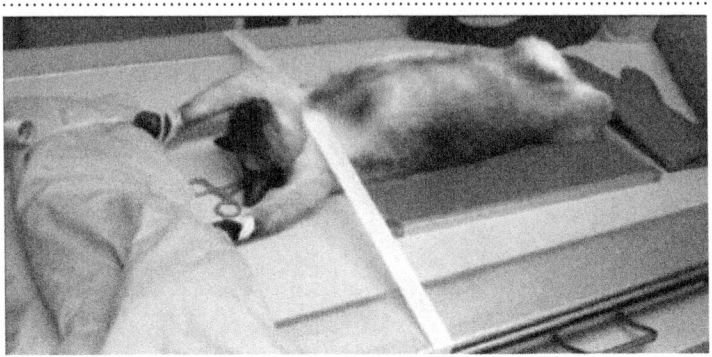

STEP 4:
This is what a properly positioned cat looks like

Neck Radiography

The principles of nonmanual restraint for neck radiography are similar in the cat and the dog. Basically, this is the same positioning for lateral thoracic radiography but the nose is elevated with a wedge and sandbags cannot be placed on the head.

STEP 1:
Place the pet in lateral recumbency and elevate the nose with a foam wedge. Tape the head to the table

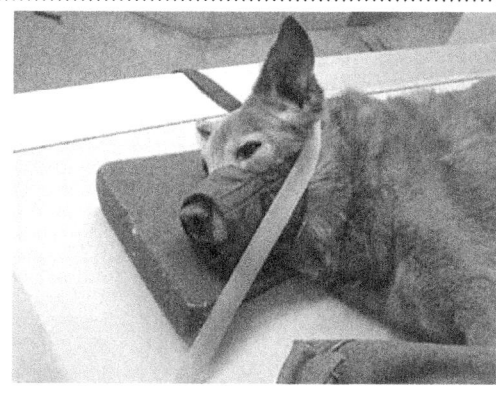

STEP 2:
Restrain the front legs using a sandbag wrapped around both feet

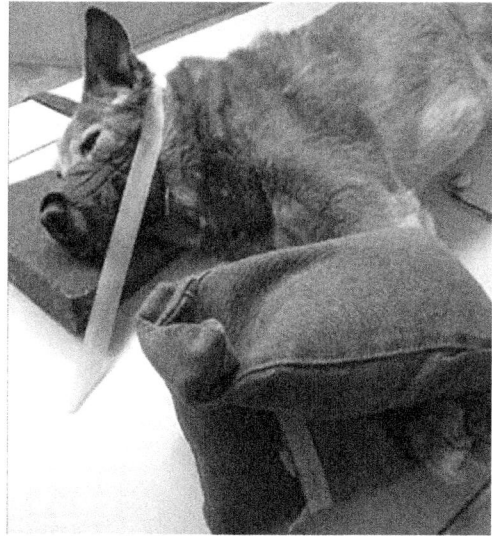

Neck Radiography - CONTINUED

STEP 3:
Restrain the hind limbs with a sandbag wrapped around the hind feet

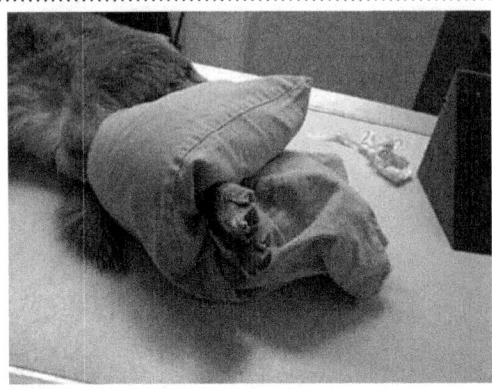

STEP 4:
The fully restrained patient

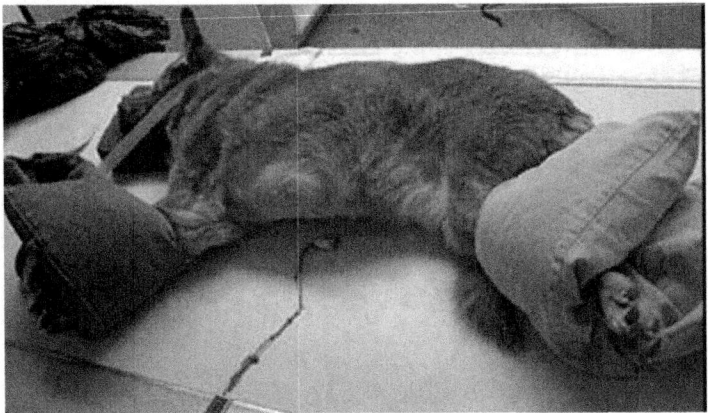

Pelvic Radiography of the Dog

The principles of pelvic radiography are similar in the cat and dog. However, with the dog, proper positioning of the pelvis is essential if the radiographs are being obtained for OFA evaluation. (Sedation is generally recommended for pelvic radiography)

STEP 1:
Position the dog in dorsal recumbency in a foam "taco" on the body and head. Additionally, apply 2 heavy laterally placed positioning devices adjacent to the shoulders

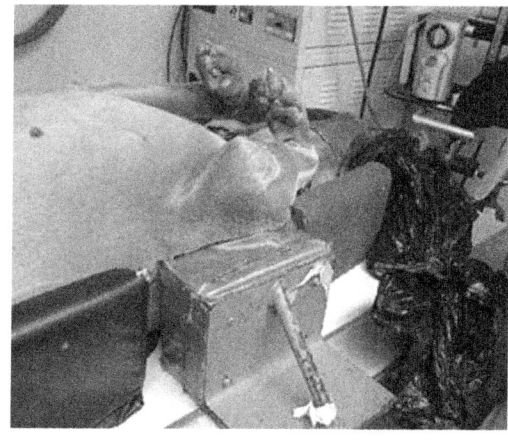

STEP 2:
Restrain the front legs with tape

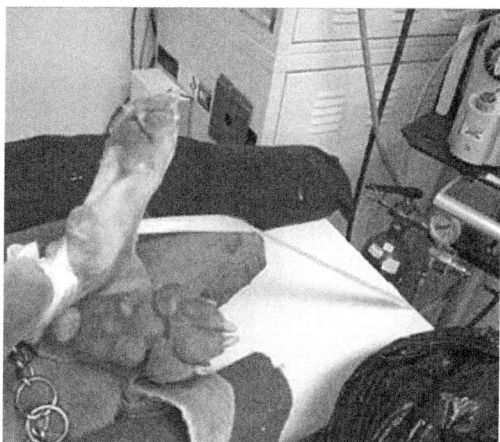

Positioning with Sandbags, Rope, and Tape

Pelvic Radiography of the Dog - CONTINUED

STEP 3:
Place a sandbag over the front legs

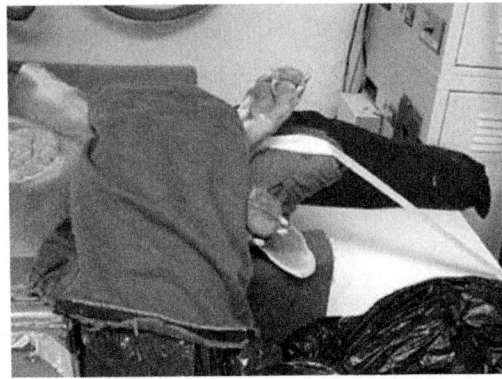

STEP 4:
Begin Positioning of the hind limbs

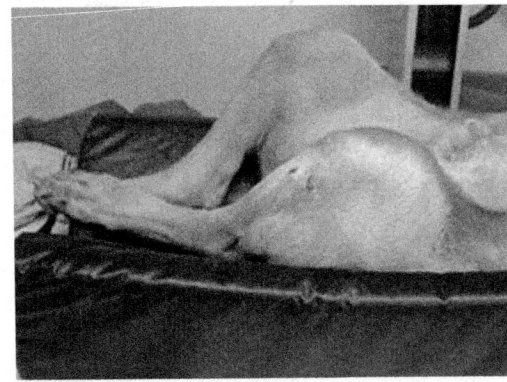

STEP 5:
Tape the stifles together

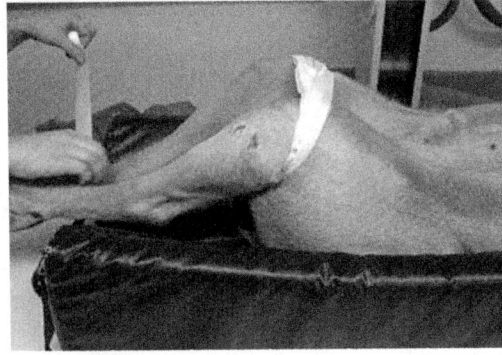

STEP 6:
Tape the right paw to the table

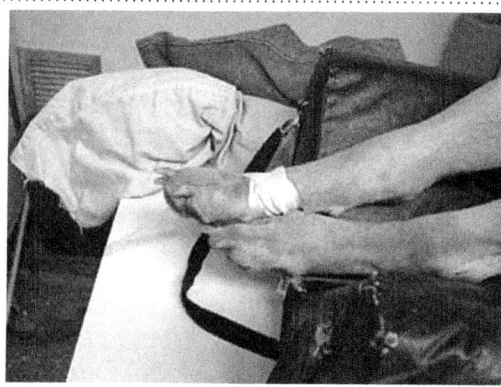

STEP 7:
Tape the left paw to the table

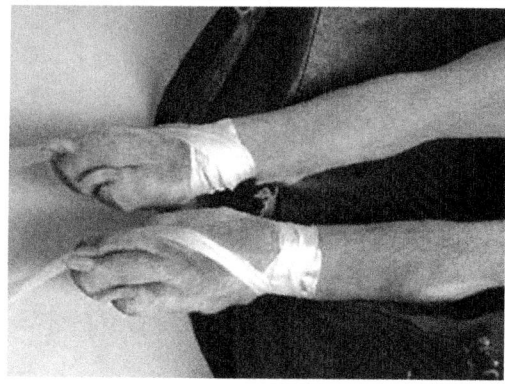

Pelvic Radiography of the Dog - CONTINUED

STEP 8:
Adjust the tape on the paws to position the limbs so that the limbs are extended and femurs are parallel.

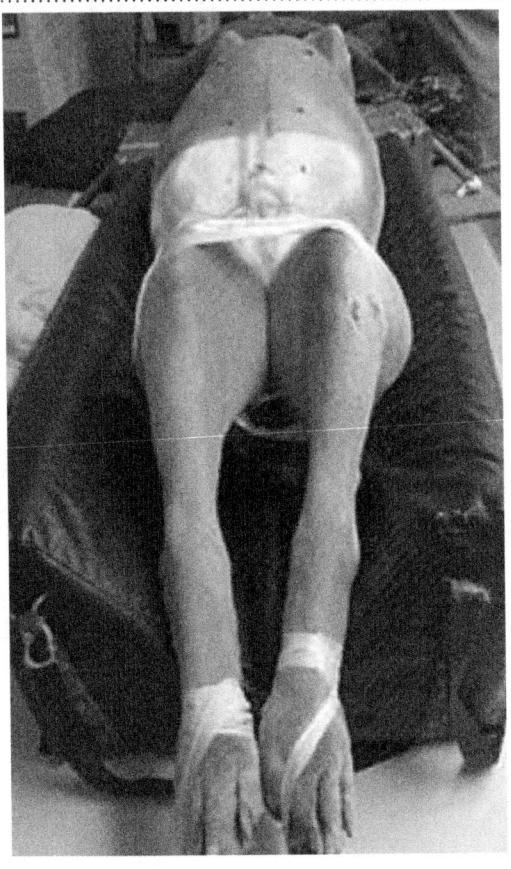

Ventral Dorsal Body and Pelvic Radiography of the Cat

The principles of pelvic radiography in the cat is similar to positioning for a ventral dorsal projection of the abdomen or thorax. Care, should be taken to properly position the hind limbs. The positioning used in these is an alternative to the technique used for positioning the cat for ventral dorsal radiography of the thorax or abdomen. In this technique we use a foam body positioner.

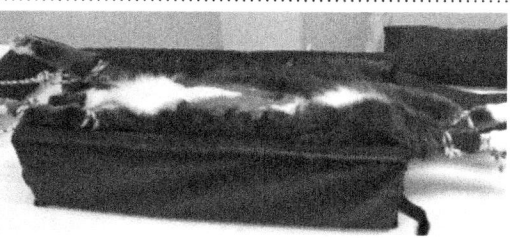

FINAL POSITION: This is what a cat that is properly positioned for pelvic radiography looks like.

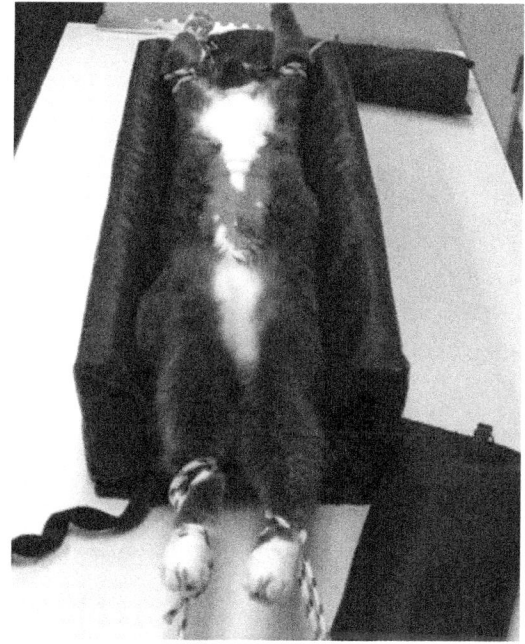

FINAL POSITION: This is another image of what a properly positoned cat looks like

Lateral Radiographs of the Dog Stifle or Tarsal Joint

STEP 1:
Secure the front legs

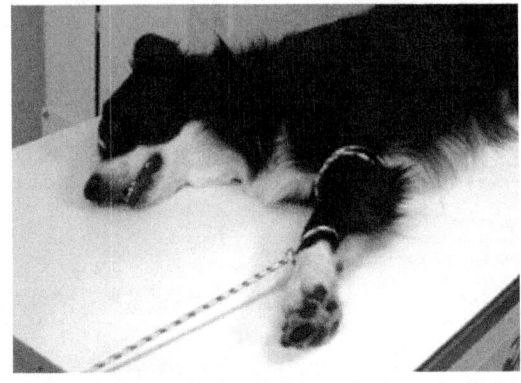

STEP 2:
Place a sandbag over the neck

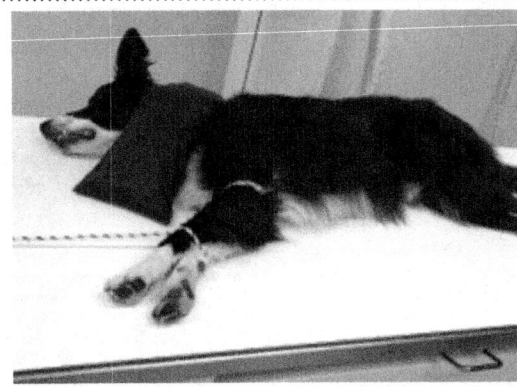

STEP 3:
Secure the top leg caudally

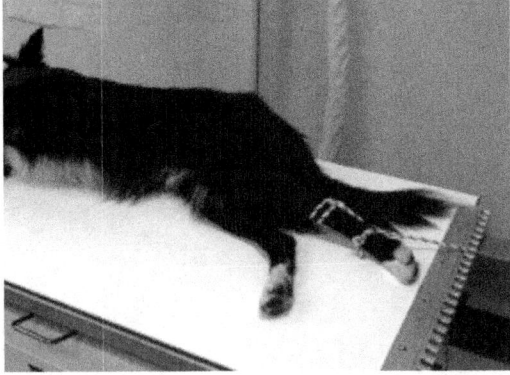

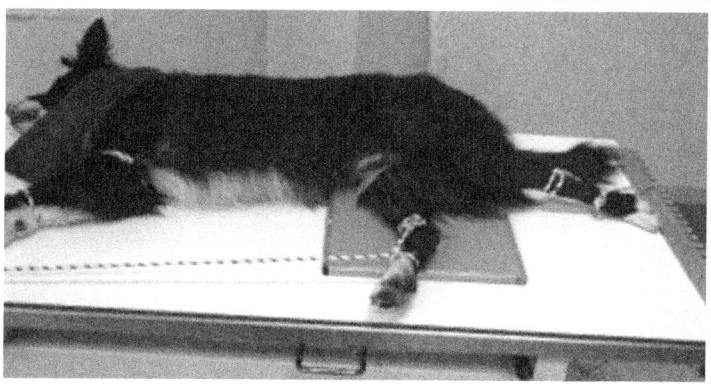

STEP 4:
Secure the bottom leg cranially and place an imaging plate under the stifle or tarsus. For dogs with heavy femoral musculature, it is recommended to place wedge sponge under the tarsus to bring the midsaggital plane on the tibia parallel to the table

Radiographs of the Cat Elbow Joint

STEP 1:
Tape or tie the back legs to the table

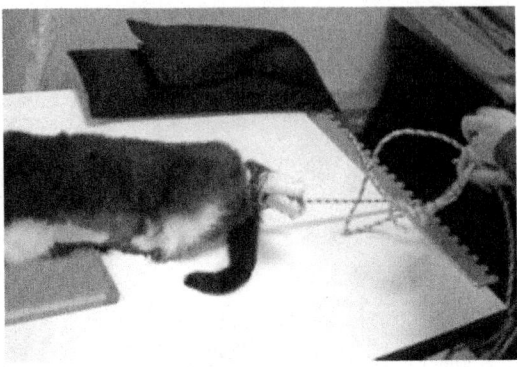

STEP 2:
Place a lead glove over the hind legs

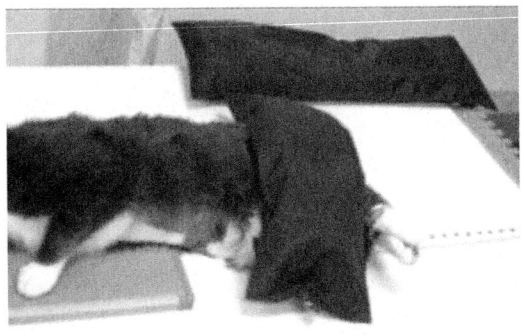

STEP 3:
Tape or tie the top leg caudally

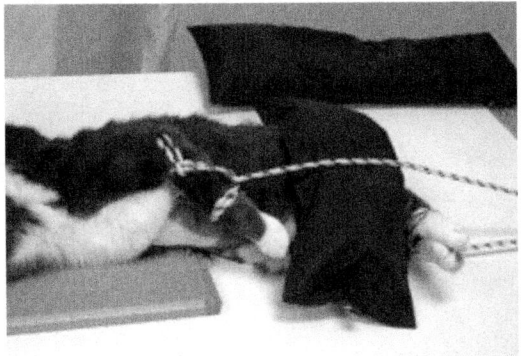

STEP 4:
Tape the limb you are radiographing to the radiographic plate. As you can see our patient is not sedated and is looking around.

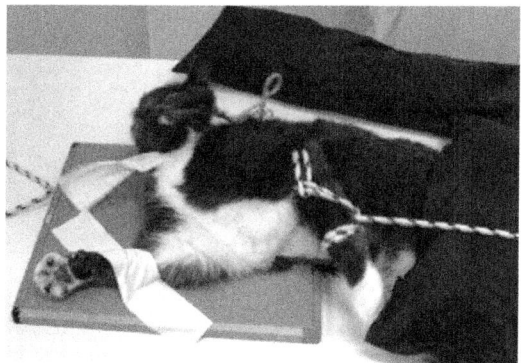

STEP 5:
Place sandbag over the patients head. This is what a properly positioned patient looks like.

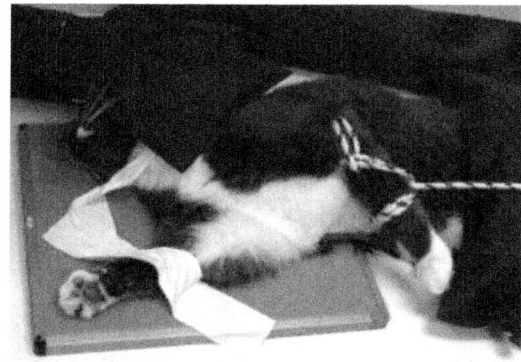

Lateral Radiographs of the Dog Elbow Joint

STEP 1:
Secure the back legs to the table.

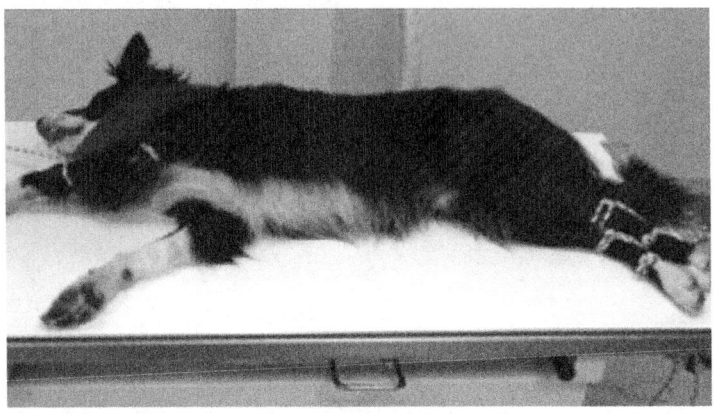

STEP 2:
Secure the upper front leg and apply a wedge to the sternum. The wedge is essential for correct positioning of the elbow.

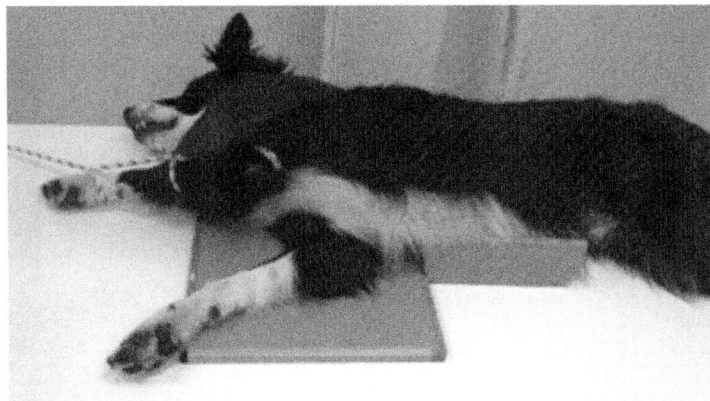

STEP 3:
Secure the bottom leg.

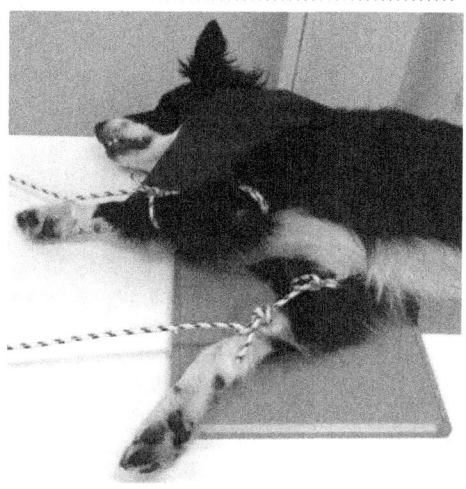

STEP 4:
Apply additional sandbags or tape as necessary to properly position the elbow. For heavily muscled dogs, it is recommended to place a small sponge under the carpus to elevate the radius/ulna to parallel to the table. This is not shown in this image.

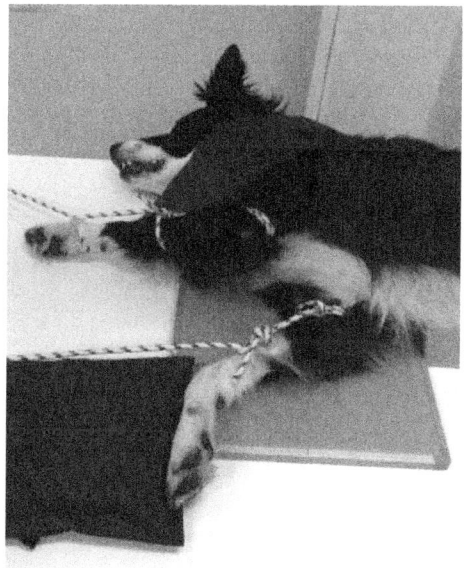

Lateral Radiographs of the Dog Carpal Joint

STEP 1:
Secure the back legs to the table.

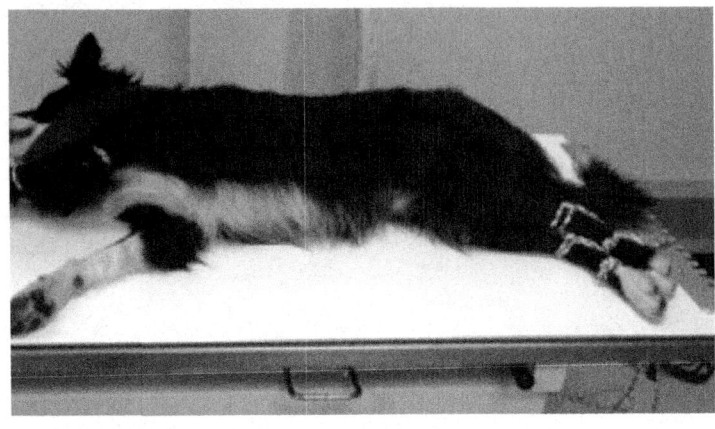

STEP 2:
Secure the upper front leg and apply a wedge to the sternum. The wedge is essential for correct positioning of the elbow.

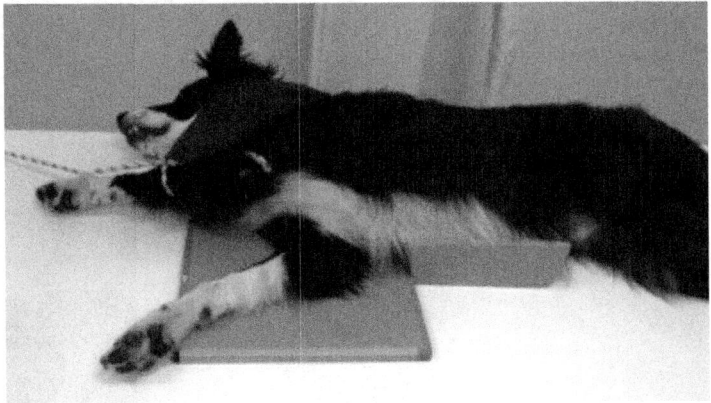

STEP 3:
Secure the bottom leg.

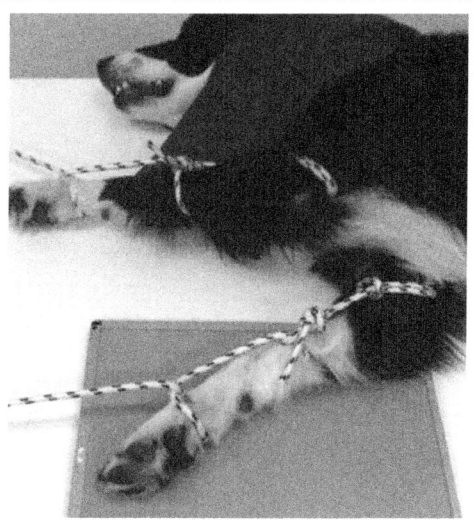

STEP 4:
Apply additional sandbags or tape as necessary to properly position the carpus.

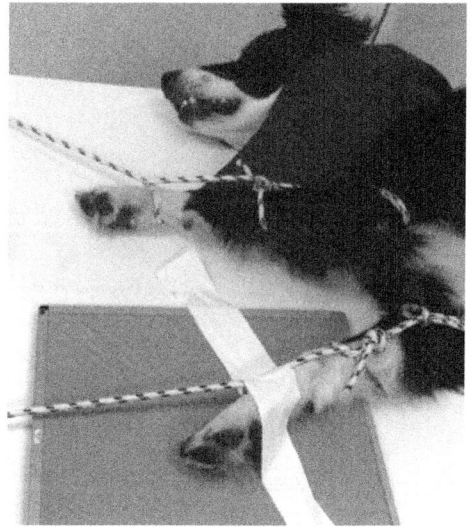

Lateral Radiographs of the Dog Shoulder Joint

STEP 1:
Secure the back legs to the table

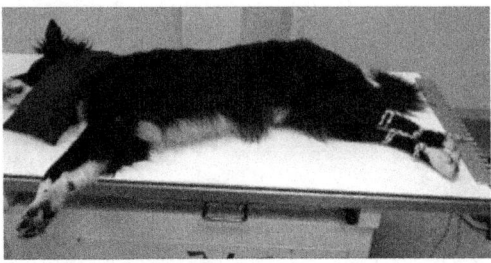

STEP 2:
Apply a large wedge to the sternum to elevate the dog (nearly) 45 degrees. Also, secure the dogs forelimb over the head. The dog should seem to be "scratching behind it's ear" when properly positioned. Don't be shy – REALLY get that leg behind the ear and be sure the elbow is elevated.

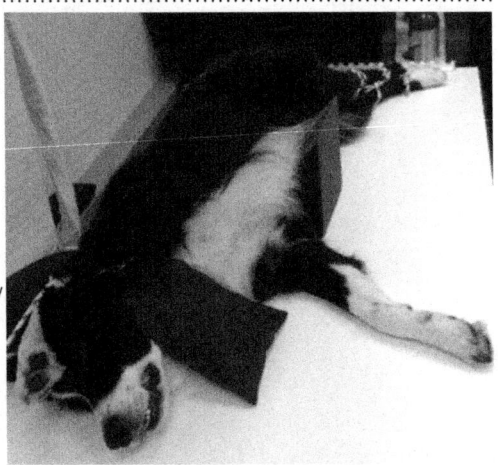

STEP 2:
This is another image of step 2. Get that leg above the head and behind the ear.

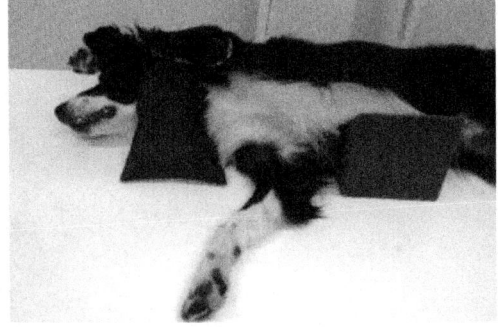

STEP 4:
Secure the front leg. Be sure to pull the elbow and paw cranially and ventrally. REALLY get that leg pulled forward toward the nose. Palpate the shoulder joints' relationship to the sternum to ensure there is no superimposition of structures.

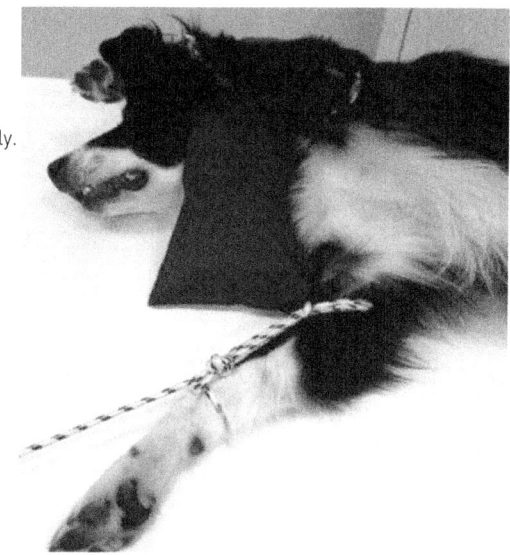

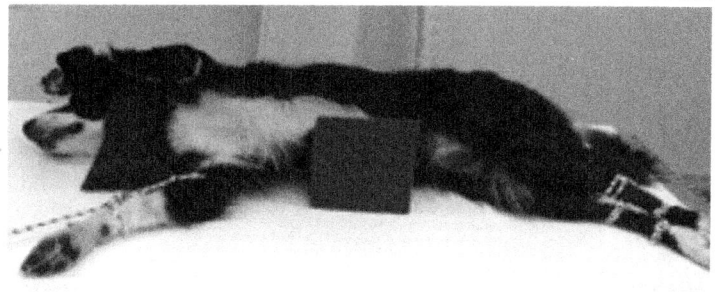

STEP 5:
This is what a properly positoned dog looks like. NOTE: most shoulder radiographs are done with a "table top" technique. Don't forget to slide a cassette under the shoulder like we did (cassette not pictured). For large breed dogs, using a bucky (i.e. grid or non-tabletop technique) is recommended.

Radiographs of the Cat Paw

It is very difficult and time consuming to radiograph the cat paw using only non-manual restraint. It is possible, but, we generally allow technicians to hold cats for radiographs of the paw. The front limb should still be tied to the table and technicians hands should never, under any circumstance be placed in the primary x-ray beam.

As you can also see in the image, the technician is standing as far away from the x-ray beam as possible.

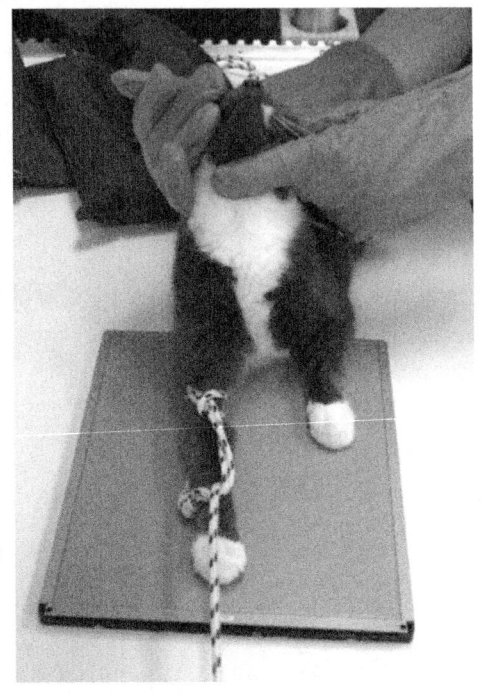

APPENDIX 1

The following is the US NRC Regulatory Guide 8.13
INSTRUCTION CONCERNING PRENATAL RADIATION
EXPOSURE

A. INTRODUCTION

8.13-8.13-1

The Code of Federal Regulations in 10 CFR Part 19, "Notices, Instructions and Reports to Workers: Inspection and Investigations," in Section 19.12, "Instructions to Workers," requires instruction in "the health protection problems associated with exposure to radiation and/or radioactive material, in precautions or procedures to minimize exposure, and in the purposes and functions of protective devices employed." The instructions must be "commensurate with potential radiological health protection problems present in the work place."

The Nuclear Regulatory Commission's (NRC's) regulations on radiation protection are specified in 10 CFR Part 20, "Standards for Protection Against Radiation"; and 10 CFR 20.1208, "Dose to an Embryo/Fetus," requires licensees to "ensure that the dose to an embryo/fetus during the entire pregnancy, due to occupational exposure of a declared pregnant woman, does not exceed 0.5 rem (5 mSv)." Section 20.1208 also requires licensees to "make efforts to avoid substantial variation above a uniform monthly exposure rate to a declared pregnant woman." A declared pregnant woman is defined in 10 CFR 20.1003 as a woman who has voluntarily informed her employer, in writing, of her pregnancy and the estimated date of conception.

This regulatory guide is intended to provide information to pregnant women, and other personnel, to help them make decisions regarding radiation exposure during pregnancy. This Regulatory Guide 8.13 supplements Regulatory Guide 8.29, "Instruction Concerning Risks from Occupational Radiation Exposure" (Ref. 1), which contains a broad discussion of the risks from exposure to ionizing radiation.

Other sections of the NRC's regulations also specify requirements for monitoring external and internal occupational dose to a declared pregnant woman. In 10 CFR 20.1502, "Conditions Requiring Individual Monitoring of External and

Internal Occupational Dose," licensees are required to monitor the occupational dose to a declared pregnant woman, using an individual monitoring device, if it is likely that the declared pregnant woman will receive, from external sources, a deep dose equivalent in excess of 0.1 rem (1 mSv). According to Paragraph (e) of 10 CFR 20.2106, "Records of Individual Monitoring Results," the licensee must maintain records of dose to an embryo/fetus if monitoring was required, and the records of dose to the embryo/fetus must be kept with the records of dose to the declared pregnant woman. The declaration of pregnancy must be kept on file, but may be maintained separately from the dose records. The licensee must retain the required form or record until the Commission terminates each pertinent license requiring the record.

The information collections in this regulatory guide are covered by the requirements of 10 CFR Parts 19 or 20, which were approved by the Office of Management and Budget, approval numbers 3150-0044 and 3150-0014, respectively. The NRC may not conduct or sponsor, and a person is not required to respond to, a collection of information unless it displays a currently valid OMB control number.

B. DISCUSSION

As discussed in Regulatory Guide 8.29 (Ref. 1), exposure to any level of radiation is assumed to carry with it a certain amount of risk. In the absence of scientific certainty regarding the relationship between low dose exposure and health effects, and as a conservative assumption for radiation protection purposes, the scientific community generally assumes that any exposure to ionizing radiation may cause undesirable biological effects and that the likelihood of these effects increases as the dose increases. At the occupational dose limit for the whole body of 5 rem (50 mSv) per year, the risk is believed to be very low.

The magnitude of risk of childhood cancer following in utero exposure is uncertain in that both negative and positive studies have been reported. The data from these studies "are consistent with a lifetime cancer risk resulting from exposure during gestation which is two to three times that for the adult" (NCRP Report No. 116, Ref. 2). The NRC has reviewed the available scientific literature and has concluded that the 0.5 rem (5 mSv) limit specified in 10 CFR 20.1208 provides an adequate margin of protection for the embryo/fetus. This dose limit reflects the desire to limit the total lifetime risk of leukemia and other cancers associated with radiation exposure during pregnancy.

In order for a pregnant worker to take advantage of the lower exposure limit and dose monitoring provisions specified in 10 CFR Part 20, the woman must declare her pregnancy in writing to the licensee. A form letter for declaring pregnancy is provided in this guide or the licensee may use its own form letter for declaring pregnancy. A separate written declaration should be submitted for each pregnancy.

C. REGULATORY POSITION

1. Who Should Receive Instruction

Female workers who require training under 10 CFR 19.12 should be provided with the information contained in this guide. In addition to the information contained in Regulatory Guide 8.29 (Ref. 1), this information may be included as part of the training required under 10 CFR 19.12.

2. Providing Instruction

The occupational worker may be given a copy of this guide with its Appendix, an explanation of the 8.13-8.13-2 contents of the guide, and an opportunity to ask questions and request additional information. The information in this guide and Appendix should also be provided to any worker or supervisor who may be affected by a declaration of pregnancy or who may have to take some action in response to such a declaration.

Classroom instruction may supplement the written information. If the licensee provides classroom instruction, the instructor should have some knowledge of the biological effects of radiation to be able to answer questions that may go beyond the information provided in this guide. Videotaped presentations may be used for classroom instruction. Regardless of whether the licensee provides classroom training, the licensee should give workers the opportunity to ask questions about information contained in this Regulatory Guide 8.13. The licensee may take credit for instruction that the worker has received within the past year at other licensed facilities or in other courses or training.

3. Licensee's Policy on Declared Pregnant Women

The instruction provided should describe the licensee's specific policy on declared pregnant women, including how those policies may affect a woman's work situation. In particular, the instruction should include a description of the licensee's policies, if any, that may affect the declared pregnant woman's work situation after she has filed a written declaration of pregnancy consistent with 10 CFR 20.1208.

The instruction should also identify who to contact for additional information as well as identify who should receive the written declaration of pregnancy. The recipient of the woman's declaration may be identified by name (e.g., John Smith), position (e.g., immediate supervisor, the radiation safety officer), or department (e.g., the personnel department).

4. Duration of Lower Dose Limits for the Embryo/Fetus

The lower dose limit for the embryo/fetus should remain in effect until the woman withdraws the declaration in writing or the woman is no longer pregnant. If a declaration of pregnancy is withdrawn, the dose limit for the embryo/fetus would apply only to the time from the estimated date of conception until the time the declaration is withdrawn. If the declaration is not withdrawn, the written declaration may be considered expired one year after submission.

5. Substantial Variations Above a Uniform Monthly Dose Rate

According to 10 CFR 20.1208(b), "The licensee shall make efforts to avoid substantial variation above a uniform monthly exposure rate to a declared pregnant woman so as to satisfy the limit in paragraph (a) of this section," that is, 0.5 rem (5 mSv) to the embryo/fetus. The National Council on Radiation Protection and Measurements (NCRP) recommends a monthly equivalent dose limit of 0.05 rem (0.5 mSv) to the embryo/fetus once the pregnancy is known (Ref. 2). In view of the NCRP recommendation, any monthly dose of less than 0.1 rem (1 mSv) may be considered as not a substantial variation above a uniform monthly dose rate and as such will not require licensee justification. However, a monthly dose greater than 0.1 rem (1 mSv) should be justified by the licensee.

8.13-8.13-3

D. IMPLEMENTATION

The purpose of this section is to provide information to licensees and applicants regarding the NRC staff's plans for using this regulatory guide.

Unless a licensee or an applicant proposes an acceptable alternative method for complying with the specified portions of the NRC's regulations, the methods described in this guide will be used by the NRC staff in the evaluation of instructions to workers on the radiation exposure of pregnant women.

REFERENCES

1. USNRC, "Instruction Concerning Risks from Occupational Radiation Exposure," Regulatory Guide 8.29, Revision 1, February 1996.
2. National Council on Radiation Protection and Measurements, Limitation of Exposure to Ionizing Radiation, NCRP Report No. 116, Bethesda, MD, 1993.

8.13-8.13-4

APPENDIX QUESTIONS AND ANSWERS CONCERNING PRENATAL RADIATION EXPOSURE

1. Why am I receiving this information?

The NRC's regulations (in 10 CFR 19.12, "Instructions to Workers") require that licensees instruct individuals working with licensed radioactive materials in radiation protection as appropriate for the situation. The instruction below describes information that occupational workers and their supervisors should know about the radiation exposure of the embryo/fetus of pregnant women.

The regulations allow a pregnant woman to decide whether she wants to formally declare her pregnancy to take advantage of lower dose limits for the embryo/fetus. This instruction provides information to help women make an informed decision whether to declare a pregnancy.

2. If I become pregnant, am I required to declare my pregnancy?

No. The choice whether to declare your pregnancy is completely voluntary. If you choose to declare your pregnancy, you must do so in writing and a lower radiation dose limit will apply to your embryo/fetus. If you choose not to declare your pregnancy, you and your embryo/fetus will continue to be subject to the same radiation dose limits that apply to other occupational workers.

3. If I declare my pregnancy in writing, what happens?

If you choose to declare your pregnancy in writing, the licensee must take measures to limit the dose to your embryo/fetus to 0.5 rem (5 millisievert) during the entire pregnancy. This is one-tenth of the dose that an occupational worker may receive in a year. If you have already received a dose exceeding 0.5 rem (5 mSv) in the period between conception and the declaration of your pregnancy, an additional dose of 0.05 rem (0.5 mSv) is allowed during the remainder of the pregnancy. In addition, 10 CFR 20.1208, "Dose to an Embryo/Fetus," requires licensees to make efforts to avoid substantial variation above a uniform monthly dose rate so that all the 0.5 rem (5 mSv) allowed dose does not occur in a short period during the pregnancy.

This may mean that, if you declare your pregnancy, the licensee may not permit you to do some of your normal job functions if those functions would have allowed you to receive more than 0.5 rem, and you may not be able to have some emergency response responsibilities.

4. Why do the regulations have a lower dose limit for the embryo/fetus of a declared pregnant woman than for a pregnant worker who has not declared?

A lower dose limit for the embryo/fetus of a declared pregnant woman is based on a consideration of greater sensitivity to radiation of the embryo/fetus and the involuntary nature of the exposure. Several scientific advisory groups have recommended (References 1 and 2) that the dose to the embryo/fetus be limited to a fraction of the occupational dose limit.

8.13-8.13-5

5. What are the potentially harmful effects of radiation exposure to my embryo/fetus?

The occurrence and severity of health effects caused by ionizing radiation are dependent upon the type and total dose of radiation received, as well as the time period over which the exposure was received. See Regulatory Guide 8.29, "Instruction Concerning Risks from Occupational Exposure" (Ref. 3), for more information. The main concern is embryo/fetal susceptibility to the harmful effects of radiation such as cancer.

6. Are there any risks of genetic defects?

Although radiation injury has been induced experimentally in rodents and insects, and in the experiments was transmitted and became manifest as hereditary disorders in their offspring, radiation has not been identified as a cause of such effect in humans. Therefore, the risk of genetic effects attributable to radiation exposure is speculative. For example, no genetic effects have been documented in any of the Japanese atomic bomb survivors, their children, or their grandchildren.

7. **What if I decide that I do not want any radiation exposure at all during my pregnancy?**

You may ask your employer for a job that does not involve any exposure at all to occupational radiation dose, but your employer is not obligated to provide you with a job involving no radiation exposure. Even if you receive no occupational exposure at all, your embryo/fetus will receive some radiation dose (on average 75 mrem (0.75 mSv)) during your pregnancy from natural background radiation.

The NRC has reviewed the available scientific literature and concluded that the 0.5 rem (5 mSv) limit provides an adequate margin of protection for the embryo/fetus. This dose limit reflects the desire to limit the total lifetime risk of leukemia and other cancers. If this dose limit is exceeded, the total lifetime risk of cancer to the embryo/fetus may increase incrementally. However, the decision on what level of risk to accept is yours. More detailed information on potential risk to the embryo/fetus from radiation exposure can be found in References 2-10.

8. **What effect will formally declaring my pregnancy have on my job status?**

Only the licensee can tell you what effect a written declaration of pregnancy will have on your job status. As part of your radiation safety training, the licensee should tell you the company's policies with respect to the job status of declared pregnant women. In addition, before you declare your pregnancy, you may want to talk to your supervisor or your radiation safety officer and ask what a declaration of pregnancy would mean specifically for you and your job status.

In many cases you can continue in your present job with no change and still meet the dose limit for the embryo/fetus. For example, most commercial power reactor workers (approximately

93%) receive, in 12 months, occupational radiation doses that are less than 0.5 rem (5 mSv) (Ref. 11). The licensee may also consider the likelihood of increased radiation exposures from accidents and abnormal events before making a decision to allow you to continue in your present job.

8.13-8.13-6

If your current work might cause the dose to your embryo/fetus to exceed 0.5 rem (5 mSv), the licensee has various options. It is possible that the licensee can and will make a reasonable accommodation that will allow you to continue performing your current job, for example, by having another qualified employee do a small part of the job that accounts for some of your radiation exposure.

9. What information must I provide in my written declaration of pregnancy?

You should provide, in writing, your name, a declaration that you are pregnant, the estimated date of conception (only the month and year need be given), and the date that you give the letter to the licensee. A form letter that you can use is included at the end of these questions and answers. You may use that letter, use a form letter the licensee has provided to you, or write your own letter.

10. To declare my pregnancy, do I have to have documented medical proof that I am pregnant?

NRC regulations do not require that you provide medical proof of your pregnancy. However, NRC regulations do not preclude the licensee from requesting medical documentation of your pregnancy, especially if a change in your duties is necessary in order to comply with the 0.5 rem (5 mSv) dose limit.

11. Can I tell the licensee orally rather than in writing that I am pregnant?

No. The regulations require that the declaration must be in writing.

12. If I have not declared my pregnancy in writing, but the licensee

suspects that I am pregnant, do the lower dose limits apply?

No. The lower dose limits for pregnant women apply only if you have declared your pregnancy in writing. The United States Supreme Court has ruled (in United Automobile Workers International Union v. Johnson Controls, Inc., 1991) that "Decisions about the welfare of future children must be left to the parents who conceive, bear, support, and raise them rather than to the employers who hire those parents" (Reference 7). The Supreme Court also ruled that your employer may not restrict you from a specific job "because of concerns about the next generation." Thus, the lower limits apply only if you choose to declare your pregnancy in writing.

13. If I am planning to become pregnant but am not yet pregnant and I inform the licensee of that in writing, do the lower dose limits apply?

No. The requirement for lower limits applies only if you declare in writing that you are already pregnant.

14. What if I have a miscarriage or find out that I am not pregnant?

If you have declared your pregnancy in writing, you should promptly inform the licensee in writing that you are no longer pregnant. However, if you have not formally declared your pregnancy in writing, you need not inform the licensee of your nonpregnant status.

15. How long is the lower dose limit in effect?

The dose to the embryo/fetus must be limited until you withdraw your declaration in writing or you 8.13-8.13-7 inform the licensee in writing that you are no longer pregnant. If the declaration is not withdrawn, the written declaration may be considered expired one year after submission.

16. If I have declared my pregnancy in writing, can I revoke my declaration of pregnancy even if I am still pregnant?

Yes, you may. The choice is entirely yours. If you revoke your declaration of pregnancy, the lower dose limit for the embryo/fetus no longer applies.

17. What if I work under contract at a licensed facility?
The regulations state that you should formally declare your pregnancy to the licensee in writing. The licensee has the responsibility to limit the dose to the embryo/fetus.

18. Where can I get additional information?
The references to this Appendix contain helpful information, especially Reference 3, NRC's Regulatory Guide 8.29, "Instruction Concerning Risks from Occupational Radiation Exposure," for general information on radiation risks. The licensee should be able to give this document to you.

For information on legal aspects, see Reference 7, "The Rock and the Hard Place: Employer Liability to Fertile or Pregnant Employees and Their Unborn Children—What Can the Employer Do?" which is an article in the journal Radiation Protection Management.

You may telephone the NRC Headquarters at (301) 415-7000. Legal questions should be directed to the Office of the General Counsel, and technical questions should be directed to the Division of Industrial and Medical Nuclear Safety.

You may also telephone the NRC Regional Offices at the following numbers: Region I, (610) 337-5000; Region II, (404) 562-4400; Region III, (630) 829-9500; and Region IV, (817) 860-8100. Legal questions should be directed to the Regional Counsel, and technical questions should be directed to the Division of Nuclear Materials Safety.

8.13-8.13-8

REFERENCES FOR APPENDIX

- National Council on Radiation Protection and Measurements, Limitation of Exposure to Ionizing Radiation, NCRP Report No. 116, Bethesda, MD, 1993.
- International Commission on Radiological Protection, 1990 Recommendations of the International Commission on Radiological Protection, ICRP Publication 60, Ann. ICRP 21: No. 1-3, Pergamon Press, Oxford, UK, 1991.

- USNRC, "Instruction Concerning Risks from Occupational Radiation Exposure," Regulatory Guide 8.29, Revision 1, February 1996.[1] (Electronically available at www.nrc.gov/NRC/RG/index.html)
- Committee on the Biological Effects of Ionizing Radiations, National Research Council, Health Effects of Exposure to Low Levels of Ionizing Radiation (BEIR V), National Academy Press, Washington, DC, 1990.
- United Nations Scientific Committee on the Effects of Atomic Radiation, Sources and Effects of Ionizing Radiation, United Nations, New York, 1993.
- R. Doll and R. Wakeford, "Risk of Childhood Cancer from Fetal Irradiation," The British Journal of Radiology, 70, 130-139, 1997.
- David Wiedis, Donald E. Jose, and Timm O. Phoebe, "The Rock and the Hard Place: Employer Liability to Fertile or Pregnant Employees and Their Unborn Children—What Can the Employer Do?" Radiation Protection Management, 11, 41-49, January/February 1994.
- National Council on Radiation Protection and Measurements, Considerations Regarding the Unintended Radiation Exposure of the Embryo, Fetus, or Nursing Child, NCRP Commentary No. 9, Bethesda, MD, 1994.
- National Council on Radiation Protection and Measurements, Risk Estimates for Radiation Protection, NCRP Report No. 115, Bethesda, MD, 1993.

---

[1]Single copies of regulatory guides, both active and draft, and draft NUREG documents may be obtained free of charge by writing the Reproduction and Distribution Services Section, OCIO, USNRC, Washington, DC 20555-0001, or by fax to(301)415-2289, or by email to DISTRIBUTION@NRC.GOV. Active guides may alsobe purchased fromthe National Technical Information Service on a standing order basis. Details on this service may be obtained

by writing NTIS, 5285 Port Royal Road, Springfield, VA 22161. Copies of active and draft guides are available for inspection or copying for a fee from the NRC Public Document Room at 2120 L Street NW., Washington, DC; the PDR's mailing address is Mail Stop LL-6, Washington, DC 20555; telephone (202)634-3273; fax (202)634-3343.

8.13-8.13-9

1. National Radiological Protection Board, Advice on Exposure to Ionising Radiation During Pregnancy, National Radiological Protection Board, Chilton, Didcot, UK, 1998.
2. M.L. Thomas and D. Hagemeyer, "Occupational Radiation Exposure at Commercial Nuclear Power Reactors and Other Facilities, 1996," Twenty-Ninth Annual Report, NUREG-0713, Vol. 18, USNRC, 1998.[22]

APPENDIX 2

Declaration of Pregnancy form

Declaration of Pregnancy (to be completed by radiation worker)

With this notice I inform you that I am pregnant or trying to become pregnant with an estimated conception date of _____ and an expected delivery date of _____. I understand the radiation exposure limit set by the Nuclear Regulatory Commission for embryo/fetus of the declared pregnant worker* is 500 mrem for the entire gestation period.

Please check the following as appropriate:

    I have questions related to the radiation protection of the embryo/fetus and would like to have the Radiation Safety Officer contact me at _____.

    I have questions related to the radiation protection of the embryo/fetus and will contact the Radiation Safety Officer at 657-278-4345.

    I do not have questions related to the radiation protection at this time. I understand that I may contact the Radiation Safety Officer if I have any questions in the future concerning this pregnancy.

Signature: _____

Date: _____

Training Documentation (to be completed by supervisor)

Supervisor (if different): _____

Telephone #: _____

Pregnancy Declaration Received (date): _____

NRC Guide 8.13 Received (date): _____

Certification

I hereby certify that I have received a copy of NRC Reg Guide 8.13, and a personal monitoring program has been established for me. I have been given an opportunity to ask questions concerning the safety aspects of exposure to the fetus.

Signature: _____

Date: _____

Signature: _____

Date: _____

Printed in Dunstable, United Kingdom